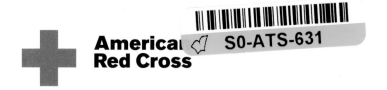

Wilderness and Remote First Aid
Emergency Reference Guide

Special thanks to the Boy Scouts of America for facilitating the task force that produced the
Wilderness First Aid Curriculum and Doctrine Guidelines.

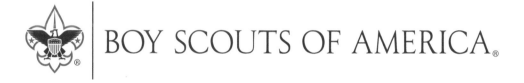

BOY SCOUTS OF AMERICA.

The following organizations provided review of the materials and/or support for the
American Red Cross Wilderness and Remote First Aid program:

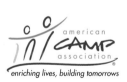

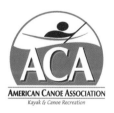

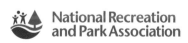

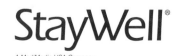

A MediMedia USA Company

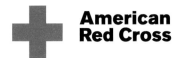

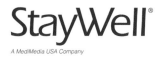

A MediMedia USA Company

Content in the *Wilderness and Remote First Aid Emergency Reference Guide* is
based on the *2010 Boy Scouts of America (BSA) Wilderness First Aid Curriculum
and Doctrine Guidelines* and reflects the 2005 Consensus on Science for CPR
and Emergency Cardiovascular Care and the 2005 Guidelines for First Aid. The
Wilderness First Aid Curriculum and Doctrine Guidelines were developed through
a task force facilitated by the BSA. The Wilderness and Remote First Aid course
carefully follows these guidelines.

The emergency care procedures outlined in this manual reflect the standard of
knowledge and accepted emergency practices in the United States at the time this
manual was published. It is the reader's responsibility to stay informed of changes
in the emergency care procedures.

Printed in the United States of America.
Printing/Binding by RR Donnelley

StayWell
780 Township Line Rd.
Yardley, PA 19067

ISBN: 978-1-58480-468-0
10 11 12 13 14 / 9 8 7 6 5 4 3 2 1

Acknowledgments

The American Red Cross Wilderness and Remote First Aid program and supporting materials were developed through the dedication of both employees and volunteers. Their commitment to excellence made this program possible.

Contents

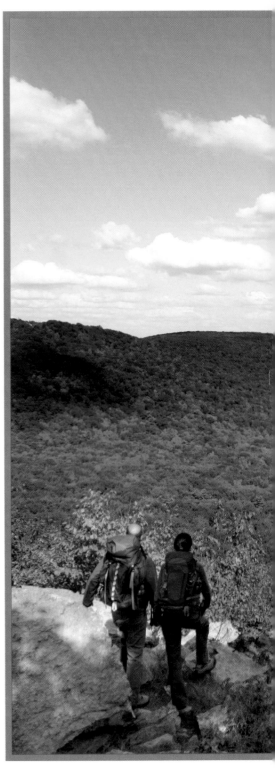

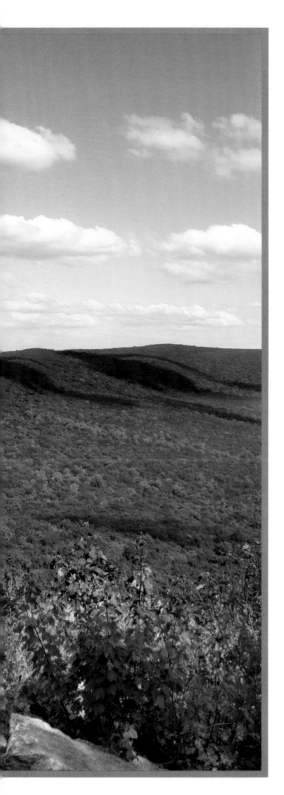

SPECIAL SITUATIONS

Photo Credits

Select Photography: Barbara Proud

Cover and Table of Contents Photography: iperdesign, Inc.

Injuries and Illnesses Section Opener: © iStockphoto.com/Arthur Carlo Franco

Special Situations Section Opener: Image Copyright robcocquyt,
2009 Used under license from Shutterstock.com

Back Cover (Man cutting down tree): © Jupiter Images Corporation

Back Cover (Rafting): Image Copyright Ron Hilton,
2009 Used under license from Shutterstock.com

Back Cover (Camping): © iStockphoto.com/Sportstock

**Many thanks to Keith Van Derzee and the YMCA Camp Ockanickon
staff for opening the camp to us and providing assistance with the
photography shoot.**

Skill
Sheets

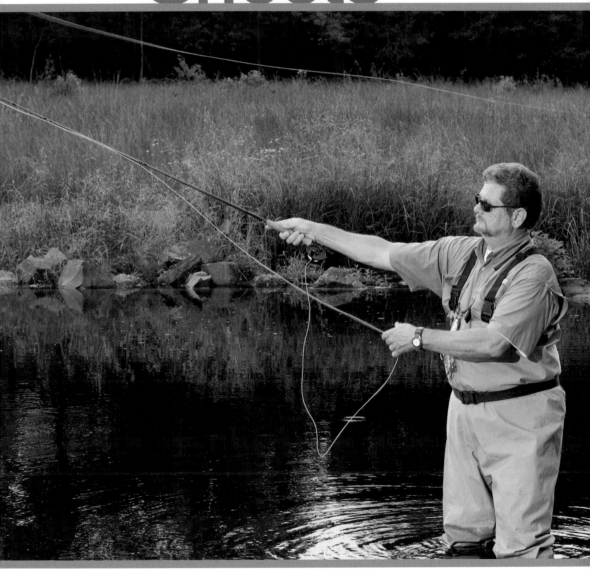

Glove Removal

NOTE To remove gloves without spreading germs, never touch your bare skin with the outside of either glove.

STEP 1

Pinch the palm side of one glove near your wrist. Carefully pull the glove off so that it is inside out.

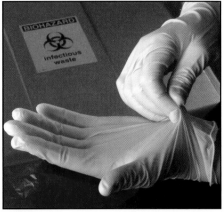

STEP 1

STEP 2

Hold the glove in the palm of your gloved hand. Slip two fingers under the glove at the wrist of the remaining gloved hand.

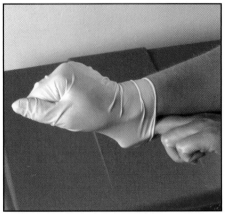

STEP 2

STEP 3

Pull the glove until it comes off, inside out. The first glove should end up *inside* the glove you just removed.

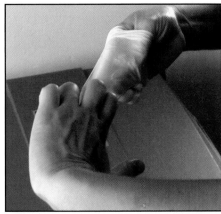

STEP 3

STEP 4

Always wash your hands after removing gloves. Use soap and running water.

<u>NOTE</u>   If soap and running water are unavailable and there is no visible matter present, rub hands thoroughly with an alcohol-based hand sanitizer.

WHAT TO DO NEXT

Always dispose of gloves and other personal protective equipment (PPE) in a proper biohazard container.

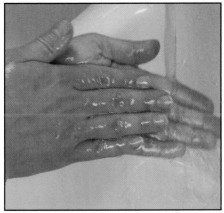

STEP 4

Checking an Unconscious Person

(APPEARS TO BE UNCONSCIOUS)

NOTE   Wear disposable gloves
and PPE.

STEP 1

CHECK scene, then **CHECK** person.

NOTE   If checking an unconscious
child, obtain consent from a
parent or guardian, if present.

STEP 2

Tap shoulder and shout, "Are
you OK?"

STEP 3

No response, **CALL 9-1-1**.

NOTE   If an unconscious person is
face-down, roll face-up,
supporting the head, neck
and back.

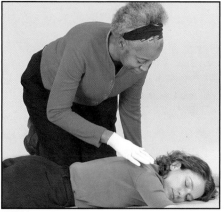

STEP 2

STEP 4

Open airway (tilt head, lift chin);
CHECK for movement and normal
breathing for no more than
10 seconds.

NOTE   Irregular, gasping or shallow
breaths are NOT effective.

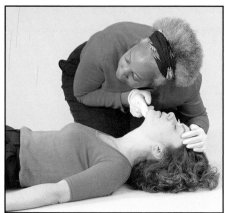

STEP 4

STEP 5

If no breathing, give **2** rescue breaths.

STEP 6

If breathing, **CHECK** for circulation. For an adult, this means checking for severe bleeding. For a child, this means checking for severe bleeding and checking for a pulse for no more than 10 seconds.

WHAT TO DO NEXT

IF BREATHING—Place in a recovery position and monitor ABCs.
IF NO BREATHING AND BREATHS GO IN (AND NO PULSE FOR A CHILD)—Get into position to perform CPR or use an AED (if AED is immediately available).

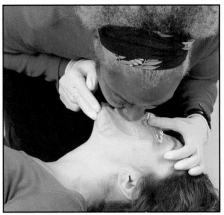

STEP 5

Conscious Choking—Adult and Child

(CANNOT COUGH, SPEAK OR BREATHE)

STEP 1

CHECK scene, then **CHECK** person.

STEP 2

Have someone **CALL 9-1-1**.

STEP 3

Obtain consent.

STEP 4

Lean the person forward and give **5** back blows with the heel of your hand.

NOTE For a child, stand or kneel behind the child, depending on his or her size.

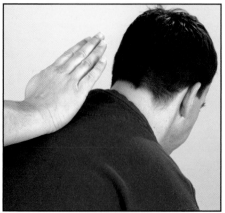

STEP 4

STEP 5

Give **5** quick, upward abdominal thrusts.

<u>NOTE</u> ■ Give chest thrusts to a choking person who is pregnant or too big for you to reach around.

■ You can give yourself abdominal thrusts by using your hands, just as you would do to another person, or lean over and press your abdomen against any firm object (e.g., the back of a chair).

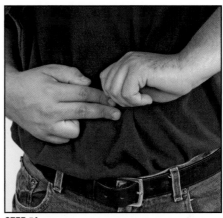

STEP 5A

STEP 6

Continue back blows and abdominal thrusts until:

■ Object is forced out.
■ Person can breathe or cough forcefully.
■ Person becomes unconscious.

WHAT TO DO NEXT

IF PERSON BECOMES UNCONSCIOUS–**CALL 9-1-1**, IF NOT ALREADY DONE, and give care for unconscious choking.

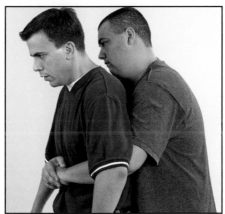

STEP 5B

CPR—Adult and Child

(NO SIGNS OF LIFE)

After checking an injured or ill person

STEP 1

Give cycles of **30** chest compressions and **2** rescue breaths.

NOTE   You can also use one hand to compress the chest of a child. If you are using one hand, place one hand on the center of the child's chest and the other hand on the child's forehead.

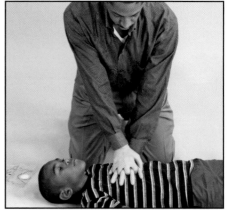

STEP 1A

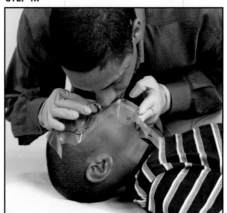

STEP 1B

STEP 2

Continue CPR until:

- Scene becomes unsafe.
- You find a sign of life.
- AED is ready to use.
- You are too exhausted to continue.
- Another trained responder arrives and takes over.

WHAT TO DO NEXT

USE AN AED AS SOON AS ONE BECOMES AVAILABLE.

Unconscious Choking—Adult and Child

(BREATHS DO NOT GO IN)

*After checking an injured or
ill person*

STEP 1

For an unconscious adult, tilt head
farther back. For an unconscious child,
retilt the child's head. Try **2** rescue
breaths again.

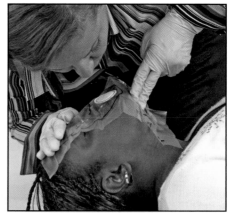

STEP 1A

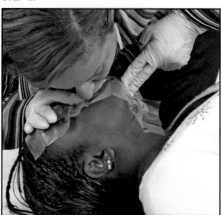

STEP 1B

STEP 2

If chest does not rise—
Give **30** chest compressions.

NOTE   Remove breathing
barrier when giving chest
compressions.

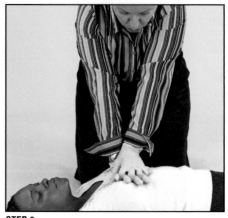

STEP 2

STEP 3

Look for an object.

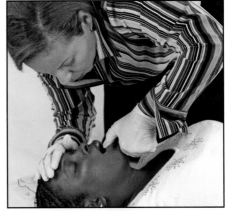

STEP 3

STEP 4

Remove if an object is seen.

NOTE For a child, remove the object with your little finger by sliding it along the inside of the cheek, using a hooking motion to sweep the object out.

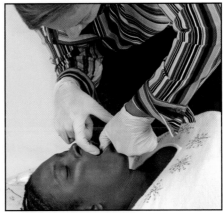

STEP 4

STEP 5

Try **2** rescue breaths.

WHAT TO DO NEXT

IF BREATHS DO NOT GO IN–
Continue Steps 2–5.
IF BREATHS GO IN–

- Check for movement and normal breathing. For an unconscious child, check for a pulse as well.
- Give care based on conditions found.

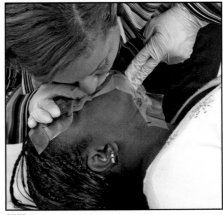

STEP 5

AED—Adult and Child

NOTE If two trained responders are present, one should perform CPR while the second responder operates the AED.

After checking an injured or ill person

(For child, ages 1 to 8 or less than 55 pounds)

STEP 1
Turn on AED.

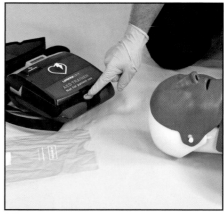

STEP 1

STEP 2
Wipe chest dry.

NOTE Remove any medication patches with a gloved hand.

STEP 3
Attach pads to bare chest.

NOTE If pediatric pads risk touching each other, use front/back pad placement.

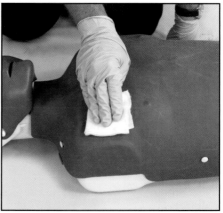

STEP 2

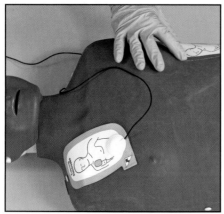

STEP 3A

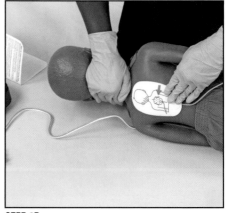

STEP 3B

STEP 4

Plug in connector, if necessary.

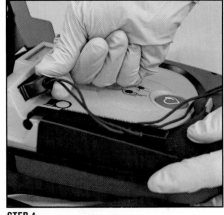

STEP 4

STEP 5

- Make sure no one, including you, is touching the person.
- Say, "EVERYONE STAND CLEAR."

STEP 6

- Push "analyze" button, if necessary.
- Let AED analyze heart rhythm.

STEP 7

IF SHOCK ADVISED—

- Make sure no one, including you, is touching the person.
- Say, "EVERYONE STAND CLEAR."
- Push "shock" button, if necessary.

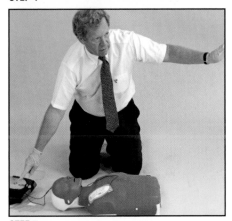

STEP 5

WHAT TO DO NEXT

AFTER SHOCK—GIVE **5** CYCLES OR ABOUT **2** MINUTES OF CPR. LET AED REANALYZE.

IF NO SHOCK ADVISED—GIVE **5** CYCLES OR ABOUT **2** MINUTES OF CPR.

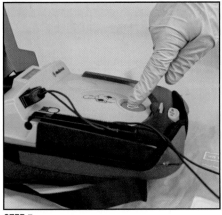

STEP 7

Injuries
and IIInesses

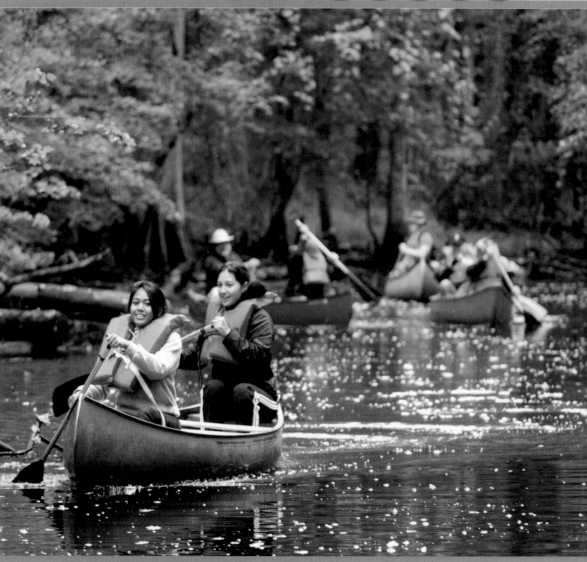

As Reflected in Boy Scouts of America *Wilderness First Aid Curriculum and Doctrine Guidelines*

Wilderness and Remote First Aid Kits

Include the following contents in personal and group wilderness and remote first aid kits (Figure 1):

Personal First Aid Kit

- Adhesive bandages (6)
- Sterile gauze pads, 3-x-3-inch (2)
- Adhesive tape (1 small roll)
- Moleskin, 3-x-6-inch (1)
- Soap (1 small bar) or alcohol-based hand sanitizing gel (1 travel-sized bottle)
- Antibiotic ointment (1 small tube)
- Scissors (1 pair)
- Non-latex disposable gloves (1 pair)
- Cardiopulmonary resuscitation (CPR) breathing barrier (1)
- Tweezers (1)
- Wilderness and Remote First Aid Report Form/Rescue Request and pencil

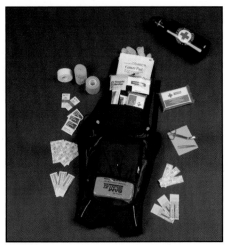

Figure 1

Group First Aid Kit

- Gauze bandage, 3-inch rolls (2)
- Self-adhesive bandage, 2-inch roll (1)
- Adhesive tape, 1-inch rolls (2)
- Alcohol pads (12)
- Povidone-iodine pads (12)
- Assorted adhesive bandages (1 box)
- Elastic bandages, 3-inch-wide (2)
- Sterile gauze pads, 4-x-4-inch (12)
- Moleskin, 3-x-6-inch (4)

- Gel pads for blisters and burns (2 packets)
- Antibiotic ointment (1 tube)
- Hydrocortisone cream 1 percent (1 tube)
- Triangular bandages (4)
- Soap (1 small bar) or alcohol-based hand sanitizing gel (1 travel-sized bottle)
- Scissors (1 pair)
- Tweezers (1 pair)
- Safety pins (12)
- Non-latex disposable gloves (6 pairs)
- Protective goggles/safety glasses (1 pair)
- CPR breathing barrier (1)
- Wilderness and Remote First Aid Report Form/Rescue Request and pencil
- Optional items:
  - Instant cold compress
  - Space blanket
  - Original size SAM® Splint

Additional Items Mentioned in Course for Consideration

- Oil of cloves (eugenol)
- Denture adhesive
- Irrigation syringe
- Thermometer
- Commercial tourniquet
- Ibuprofen
- Children's chewable aspirin (81 mg)
- Acetaminophen
- Oral antihistamine
- Properly labeled prescription medications for individuals (e.g., EpiPen®, nitroglycerin, high-altitude drugs)
- Needle
- Alcohol (and/or vinegar)
- Tampons/pads
- Decongestant nasal spray
- Over-the-counter diarrhea medication

- Zinc oxide powder
- Chemical heat packs

NOTE The patient should only take medication if he or she can swallow and has no known contraindications. Patients should read and follow all label or health care provider instructions. Check state and local regulations regarding use of prescription and over-the-counter medications. Aspirin and products containing aspirin should not be given to a child younger than 19 years of age if he or she has a fever-causing illness.

Other Important Items That Are Useful in First Aid and Other Emergencies

- Full water bottle(s) (especially in waterless areas)
- Water purification and backup
- Ground insulation (e.g., a "sit-upon" camp mat)
- Shelter (could be a plastic tube shelter)
- SAM® Splint
- Plastic bag
- Emergency blanket
- Signaling device (e.g., mirror, whistle)
- Duct tape
- Identification/medical form
- Special environmental essentials (e.g., ice axe, cold weather sailing gear)

NOTE No piece of equipment is as valuable as the person who uses it.

⊘ CHECK ⊙ CALL ♥ CARE
for the Wilderness

If you find yourself in an emergency, you should follow three basic emergency action principles: **CHECK–CALL–CARE**. These principles will help guide you in caring for the patient and will help ensure your own safety.

⊘ CHECK:
CHECK the Scene, the Resources and the Person

CHECK the Scene

- Establish control and recognize the emergency.
- CHECK the scene before you approach to make sure it is safe for you, the person, other members of the group and any bystanders.
- Follow standard precautions to prevent disease transmission.
- Obtain consent from a conscious patient or, if a minor, from the parent or guardian. If the patient is unconscious, consent is implied.
- CHECK for clues about the mechanism of injury (MOI) or nature of the illness.
- Move the patient only if necessary to prevent additional harm.

> **NOTE** If the scene is not safe and there is a way to call for additional help, do so quickly. Be ready to continue checking and caring for the patient if the scene becomes safe.

CHECK the Resources

- Identify available resources, including materials and additional trained responders.

CHECK the Patient
Primary (Initial) Assessment

Use the ABCDEs to assess life-threatening conditions.

- **A** = If the patient is unconscious, use the head-tilt/chin-lift technique to open the **airway** (Figure 1). A patient who is speaking or breathing has an open airway, but ask if he or she is having problems breathing.

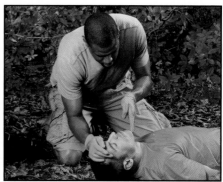

Figure 1

- **B** = Look, listen and feel for movement, normal **breathing** and quality of **breathing** (for no more than 10 seconds) (Figure 2). If the patient is not breathing, immediately begin rescue breathing or cardiopulmonary resuscitation (CPR).

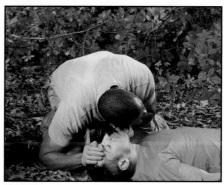

Figure 2

- **C** = Assess the patient's **circulation.** Check for a pulse in a child (for no more than 10 seconds or for up to 45 seconds for a hypothermic child). For an adult and child, scan for severe bleeding. If the patient does not have a pulse, immediately begin CPR. If severely bleeding, immediately expose the wound and use direct pressure to control the bleeding.

- **D** = Look for any **disability** as a result of damage to the spinal cord. If you suspect a spinal injury, keep a hand on the patient's head or ask someone else to take control of the patient's head.
- **E** = Check for **exposure** to injuries caused by extreme environmental conditions. Protect the patient from extreme conditions. Expose skin to assess and care for wounds. Cover skin after assessing and caring for wounds.

If you find a life-threatening condition during the primary assessment, CALL for help if possible and give CARE for the condition found. The caller should be prepared with information about the patient, location/environment and resources (people and materials). If you do not find a life-threatening condition, continue to the secondary assessment and SAMPLE history before giving specific care for an injury or illness.

Secondary (Focused) Assessment

Hands-On Physical Exam

Check the patient head to toe during the hands-on physical exam, going in the following order: head, face, ears, neck, chest, abdomen, pelvis, genitalia, each arm, each leg and back.
- Look for DOTS:
  - D = Deformity
  - O = Open injuries
  - T = Tenderness
  - S = Swelling
- Check circulation, sensation and motion (CSM) at each extremity.
- Assess skin color, temperature and moisture.

Level of Responsiveness

Use AVPU to describe the patient's level of responsiveness (LOR). LOR can also be referred to as level of consciousness (LOC).
- **A = Alert** and able to answer orientation questions
  - *A+O×4:* knows who (name), where (current location), when (day) and what happened
  - *A+O×3:* knows who, where and when
  - *A+O×2:* knows only who and where
  - *A+O×1:* knows only who

- **V** = Responds only to **verbal** stimuli (e.g., by grimacing or rolling away from your voice when you speak or shout)
- **P** = Responds only to **painful** stimuli (e.g., pinch)
- **U** = **Unresponsive** to any stimuli

Normal Vital Signs for an Adult

- Respiratory rate (breath): 12 to 20 breaths per minute; regular and unlabored pace
- Heart rate (pulse): 50 to 100 beats per minute; strong and regular
- Skin color, temperature and moisture: pink, warm and dry to the touch

SAMPLE History

Use the SAMPLE history to gain essential information about the patient's medical history. Ask the patient questions, such as those listed below, and record the answers on the Wilderness and Remote First Aid Report Form/Rescue Request:

- **S = Signs and symptoms.** What are your signs and symptoms (i.e., what hurts)? How do you feel? Are you experiencing any pain, nausea, light-headedness or other things that are not visible?
- **A = Allergies.** Do you have any known allergies or allergic reactions? What happens? Has there been any recent exposure?
- **M = Medications.** What medications are you taking? Are they over-the-counter or prescription? What is the medication for? When was it last taken? Can you tell me where the medication is so we can keep it with you?
- **P = Pertinent past medical history.** Has anything like this happened before? Are you currently under a health care provider's care for anything? Could you be pregnant (if a woman)?
- **L = Last intake and output.** When did you last eat or drink? How much? Are you cold, hungry or exhausted? When did you last urinate and defecate? Were they normal?
- **E = Events leading up to the injury or illness.** What led up to the incident? When did it happen? How did it happen, in order of occurrence?

It is often appropriate for the leader of a wilderness group to travel with a health history for each participant. Those forms, frequently combined with consent for treatment, may provide useful information to emergency response personnel and aid in collecting the SAMPLE history. However, each step in the SAMPLE history still must be asked, even if such forms are available for reference.

⊚ CALLing for Help:
Stay or Go, Fast or Slow

Being in the wilderness or remote setting makes CALLing important to everyone involved. Ideally, immediate verbal communication is available by phone or radio to predetermined emergency agencies. Primary and backup communication procedures should be established prior to a remote trip. Such procedures could include sending members of the party to the closest area where a signal can be established or to the closest phone.

If advanced care is delayed, a decision to stay or to evacuate must be made. If the decision is to stay, continue CARE as trained and as needed. If evacuation is necessary, determine if it should be fast or slow. Implement a pre-trip plan using available resources. Throughout the evacuation, continue CARE as trained until the injury or illness is resolved or other help arrives.

⊚ CARE

CARE for the conditions found, prioritizing care by the severity of the injury or illness.

> **NOTE**   For more information on evacuation guidelines and care, go to the specific injury or illness in this guide.

Abdominal Problems

Abdominal pain and discomfort is a common problem in the wilderness. It ranges from mild to life threatening. You may never know the source of the problem, but you must be able to manage mild situations and know when a problem is serious enough to require evacuation.

Stomachache

⊘ When **CHECK**ing the patient, look, listen and feel for:
- Gradually increasing, widespread abdominal discomfort, often worse in the lower abdomen.
- Cramping that comes and goes.
- Nausea and vomiting.
- Diarrhea.

⊙ To give **CARE**:
- Keep the patient well hydrated.
- Give the patient a bland diet, if he or she is not vomiting.
- Maintain good personal and group hygiene.

Diarrhea

⊘ When **CHECK**ing the patient, look, listen and feel for:
- Frequent loose, watery stools.
- Presence of gastroenteritis (stomach flu).

⊙ To give **CARE**:
For mild diarrhea:
- Give the patient water or diluted, clear, non-citrus fruit juices or sports drinks.
- If the patient is not vomiting, he or she can eat rice, grains, bananas and oats, or other bland diet items.
- Avoid fats, dairy products, caffeine and alcohol.

For persistent diarrhea:

- Replace electrolytes lost in the stool using oral rehydration solutions.
  - Add 1 teaspoon of salt and 8 teaspoons of sugar to a quart of water.
  - Have the patient drink about ¼ of the solution every hour, along with as much water as tolerated.
- Use over-the-counter medication for watery diarrhea, if available.

> **NOTE** The patient should only take medication if he or she can swallow and has no known contraindications. Patients should read and follow all label or health care provider instructions. Check state and local regulations regarding use of prescription and over-the-counter medications.

- Have the patient avoid fats, dairy products, caffeine and alcohol.
- If the patient is not vomiting, allow him or her to eat rice, grains, bananas and potatoes, or other bland diet items.

Serious Abdominal Pain

⊘ When CHECKing the patient, look, listen and feel for:

- A fever higher than 102° F, which may present itself as chills or shivers.
- Persistent and/or constant pain lasting more than 12 hours.
- Pain in a specific part of the abdomen, especially if the patient guards the painful area.
- Tenderness, abdominal rigidity (stiffness) and/or distention (swelling).
- Pain that increases with movement, jarring or when putting a foot down while walking.
- Blood in vomit, feces or urine.
  - In vomit, blood looks like coffee grounds.
  - In feces, blood may be black, like tar.
  - In urine, blood is reddish color.
- Nausea, vomiting and/or diarrhea that persists for longer than 24 hours, especially if the patient is unable to stay well hydrated.
- Pain associated with the signs and symptoms of pregnancy.
- Vaginal bleeding.
- Pain associated with the signs and symptoms of shock.

To give CARE:

- Manage ABCDEs.
  - Watch and care for shock.
- Give nothing by mouth, unless evacuation will be delayed by more than a few hours, in which case give only small sips of water or ice chips, if tolerated.

Evacuation

- Evacuate slowly–**GO SLOW**–anyone with persistent abdominal discomfort.
- Evacuate rapidly–**GO FAST**–anyone with signs and symptoms of a serious abdominal problem.

Allergies and Anaphylaxis

When the body recognizes an allergen, a foreign substance that causes an allergic reaction, its immune system releases histamines and other chemicals for protection. An allergic reaction happens when the body produces too much of these substances. Allergic reactions can be mild and non-life-threatening, such as itchy skin and a stuffy nose. However, a severe allergic reaction, called *anaphylaxis,* is life threatening and must be treated immediately or the person will die.

Non-Life-Threatening Allergic Reactions

When **CHECK**ing the patient, look, listen and feel for:

- Stuffy nose/congestion.
- Flushed and itchy skin.
- Sneezing.
- Nasal discharge.
- Itchy and watery eyes.
- Swelling at a bite site.
- Hives (Figure 1).

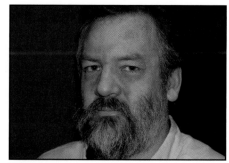

Figure 1

⊕ To give CARE:

- Remove the allergen (e.g., bees, food) or move the patient away from the allergen.
- If the person can swallow and has no known contraindications, help the patient self-administer an antihistamine.

> **NOTE** The patient should only take medication if he or she can swallow and has no known contraindications. Patients should read and follow all label or health care provider instructions. Check state and local regulations regarding use of prescription and over-the-counter medications.

Anaphylaxis

Signs and symptoms can appear in as few as 5 minutes and most often within 45 minutes to 1 hour. The only way to reverse anaphylaxis is by immediately injecting the person with epinephrine, which reverses the overproduction of histamines. Two injectable epinephrine systems are available commercially, by prescription only, in spring-loaded syringes that function when pressed into the thigh (Figure 2). They are the EpiPen® (includes one dose) and Twinject® (includes two doses).

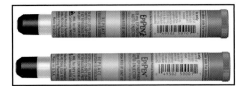

Figure 2

⊘ When CHECKing the patient, look, listen and feel for:

- In some cases, signs and symptoms of a non-life-threatening allergic reaction followed by shock.
- In most cases:
  - Extreme trouble breathing.
  - Wheezing.
  - Redness of the skin or hives.
  - Inability to speak at all or only in one- or two-word clusters.
  - Swelling of the face, lips, tongue and sometimes hands and feet.

♥ To give CARE:

- Keep everyone calm.
- Look for a medical identification (ID) tag or bracelet that may warn of a severe allergy or indicate that the patient has been prescribed an auto-injector (Figure 3).
- Try to determine whether the substance that triggered the allergic reaction is still present and if the reaction is likely to happen again.
  - Remove the allergen or move the person away from the allergen.

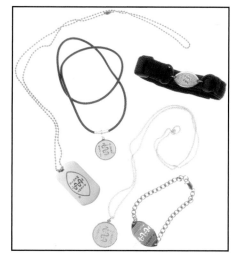

Figure 3

- Help the patient self-administer an injection of epinephrine, if necessary.
- Repeat the injection if the first one fails or the signs and symptoms return.
- Keep the patient well hydrated.
- After injection of epinephrine, if the patient has no known contraindications and can breathe and swallow, help the patient self-administer an oral antihistamine, following the directions on the label.

NOTE
- The patient should only take medication if he or she can swallow and has no known contraindications. Patients should read and follow all label or health care provider instructions. Check state and local regulations regarding use of prescription and over-the-counter medications.
- Make sure you and any others in the group know if a person in the group has allergies and carries an EpiPen® or Twinject® and where the person carries his or her EpiPen® or Twinject®.

- If using an EpiPen®:
  - Check the label to confirm that the prescription of the auto-injector is for this patient.
  - Check the expiration date of the auto-injector. If it has expired, DO NOT use it. If the medication is visible, confirm that the liquid is clear and not cloudy. If it is cloudy, DO NOT use it.

- Locate the outside middle of one thigh to use as the injection site (Figure 4).
- Grasp the auto-injector firmly in your fist, and pull off the safety cap with your other hand (Figure 5).
- Hold the (black) tip (needle end) near the patient's outer thigh so that the auto-injector is at a 90-degree angle to the thigh (Figure 6). Do not place your thumb over the end.
- Quickly and firmly push the tip straight into the outer thigh (it will go through light clothing). You will hear a click.
- Hold the auto-injector firmly in place for 10 seconds, then remove it from the thigh and massage the injection site for several seconds (Figure 7).
- Give the used auto-injector to more advanced medical personnel when they arrive.

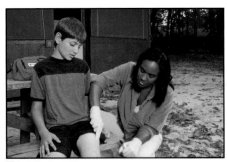

Figure 4

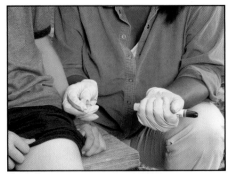

Figure 5

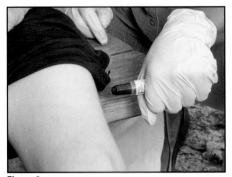

Figure 6

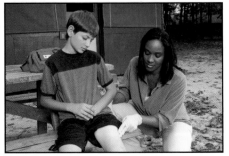

Figure 7

- If using Twinject®:
  - Remove the device from the hard case.
  - Remove the green cap, labeled 1 (Figure 8). You will see a red tip. Do not put your thumb, finger or hand over the red tip.
  - Remove the green cap, labeled 2.
  - Place the red tip against the middle of the outer thigh, press down hard until the needle enters the thigh (it will go through light clothing), and hold for a count of 10 (Figure 9).
  - Remove the Twinject® from the thigh. Check the rounded, red tip. If the needle is exposed, the dose was given.

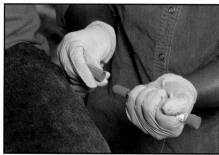

Figure 8

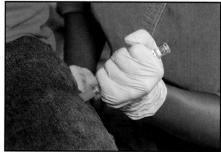

Figure 9

NOTE Only a patient should self-administer the second dose included with the Twinject® injector.

- If you need a second injection, unscrew and remove the red tip, carefully avoiding the needle.
- Grab the blue plastic and remove the syringe from the barrel.
- Remove the yellow collar from the syringe.
- Push the needle into the thigh and depress the plunger all the way to inject the second dose.
- Store the used syringe, needle first, in the hard case.

NOTE ■ Recheck the patient's airway, breathing and circulation and observe his or her response to the epinephrine.

■ A patient's breathing and heart rate are typically higher after a dose of epinephrine and the patient may also be restless.

■ Be aware that EpiPen® auto-injectors only provide one dose.

◉ CALLing for Help: Guidelines for Evacuation

- Non-life-threatening reactions that can be managed in the field do not require evacuation.
- Evacuate rapidly–**GO FAST**–anyone treated for or suffering from anaphylaxis. During evacuation, the patient should be well hydrated and kept on a regimen of oral antihistamines.

Altitude Illnesses

Altitude illnesses occur when people at a high altitude do not have enough oxygen in their blood because the air pressure is too low. The three altitude illnesses most likely to develop in the wilderness are acute mountain sickness (AMS), high altitude cerebral edema (HACE) and high altitude pulmonary edema (HAPE).

Acute Mountain Sickness

AMS commonly occurs in a person who has recently reached an altitude of around 6500 to 8000 feet. If signs and symptoms of AMS appear at lower altitudes, they are probably the result of another condition, such as dehydration or heat illness. If untreated, AMS may progress to HACE or HAPE, which is more severe.

⊘ When CHECKing the patient, look, listen and feel for:

- Someone who has recently arrived at an altitude of around 6500 to 8000 feet or more.
- Headache.
- Loss of normal appetite.
- Nausea, with or without vomiting.
- Insomnia.
- Lassitude (unusual weariness or exhaustion).

♡ To give CARE:

- Descend (go down) to a lower altitude or stop ascending (going up) and wait for improvement before going higher.
- Administer oxygen if available and you are trained to do so. This is especially helpful during sleep.

- Help the patient self-administer recommended dosages of aspirin or acetaminophen for headaches (if the patient is able to swallow and has no known contraindications).
- Care for the illness, not just the symptoms.
  - If prescribed and recommended by the patient's health care provider, help the patient self-administer medication for altitude illness (e.g., acetazolamide, dexamethasone) based on label instructions.
  - Many patients with AMS usually respond to these medications within 12 to 24 hours.

NOTE The patient should only take medication if he or she can swallow and has no known contraindications. Patients should read and follow all label or health care provider instructions. Check state and local regulations regarding use of prescription and over-the-counter medications. Anyone going to an altitude greater than around 6500 to 8000 feet should discuss this with his or her personal health care provider.

High Altitude Cerebral Edema

HACE is caused by swelling of brain tissue, which increases pressure on the brain until it fails to function properly, eventually resulting in death.

When CHECKing the patient, look, listen and feel for:

- Loss of coordination (ataxia).
  - Inability to walk a straight line or stand straight with feet together and eyes closed
- Severe headache that is not relieved by rest and medication.
- Bizarre changes in personality.
- Possible seizures and/or coma.

To give CARE:

- Descend (go down) to a lower altitude as soon as possible.
- Administer oxygen if available and you are trained to do so.
- Keep the patient from getting chilled or overheated. Cold temperatures put more pressure on the respiratory system.
- If prescribed and recommended by the patient's health care provider, help the patient self-administer medication for altitude illness (e.g., acetazolamide, dexamethasone) based on label instructions.

■ Use a portable hyperbaric chamber if available and you are trained to do so (Figure 1). DO NOT use a portable hyperbaric chamber instead of descending. Moving to a lower altitude is the only definitive care for the severely ill patient.

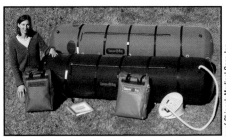

Figure 1

Courtesy of Chinook Medical Gear, Inc.

NOTE   The patient should only take medication if he or she can swallow and has no known contraindications. Patients should read and follow all label or health care provider instructions. Check state and local regulations regarding use of prescription and over-the-counter medications. Anyone going to an altitude greater than around 6500 to 8000 feet should discuss this with his or her personal health care provider.

High Altitude Pulmonary Edema

HAPE is caused by fluid collecting in the air spaces of the lungs. If enough fluid collects, the person cannot breathe adequately, and death may result.

When CHECKing the patient, look, listen and feel for:

■ Dry cough, soon followed by shortness of breath, even at rest.
■ Shortness of breath that becomes more pronounced.
■ Possible chest pain.
■ Cough that becomes more productive, first producing frothy sputum, later producing reddish sputum.

To give CARE:

■ Descend (go down) to a lower altitude as soon as possible. A descent of 1000 to 1500 feet may produce remarkable results.
■ Keep the patient from becoming chilled or overheated. Cold temperatures put more pressure on the respiratory system, particularly in HAPE.
■ Administer oxygen if available and you are trained to do so.
■ Use a portable hyperbaric chamber, if available and you are trained to do so. DO NOT use a portable hyperbaric chamber instead of descending. Moving to a lower altitude is the only definitive care for severely ill patient.

⊙ CALLing for Help: Guidelines for Evacuation

- Stopping the ascent, descending and evacuation must be considered.
- A patient with AMS should stop ascending until the signs and symptoms resolve.
- A patient with AMS does not need to evacuate unless the signs and symptoms do not resolve. If the illness does not resolve or it gets worse, descent is mandatory.
- Evacuate rapidly—**GO FAST**—to a lower altitude (descend at least 1000 to 1500 feet) anyone with HACE or HAPE.
  - Anyone with HACE or HAPE must be evaluated as soon as possible by a health care provider once a lower altitude has been reached.

Bone and Joint Injuries

There are four main types of bone and joint injuries:
- Strains: overstretched muscles and/or tendons that attach muscles to bones
- Sprains: injuries to ligaments that hold bones together at joints
- Fractures: a break, chip or crack in a bone
- Dislocations: movement of a bone away from its normal position at a joint

Because these injuries can look alike, you may have difficulty determining exactly which type of injury has occurred. This should not be a problem because in most cases, the care you give will be the same.

General Considerations

⊘ When CHECKing the patient, look, listen and feel for:

- Deformity, open injuries, tenderness and swelling (DOTS).
- Moderate or severe pain or discomfort.
- Bruising (may take hours to appear).
- Inability to move or use the affected body part normally.
- Broken bone or bone fragments sticking out of a wound.
- Feeling of bones grating or the sound of bones grating.
- Feeling or hearing of a snap or pop at the time of injury.
- Loss of circulation, sensation and motion (CSM) beyond the site of the injury, including tingling, cold or bluish color.
- Cause of injury (e.g., a fall), that suggests the injury may be severe.

⊚ To give **CARE**:

- Determine if the patient can use the injured body part.
- Have the patient rest and relax.
- Carefully remove clothing to look at the injury site if the area is not already exposed.
- Ask how the injury happened and if there are any painful areas. (High-speed impacts cause more damage than low-speed impacts.)
- Visually inspect the entire body from head to toe. Compare the two sides of the body, then carefully check each body part.
- Notice if the patient can easily move the injured part or if he or she guards it to prevent movement.
- Give care using the RICE method:
  - **R** = Have the patient **rest** the injured area and avoid any movement that causes pain.
  - **I** = **Immobilize** the injured area. For sprains and strains, wrap the injured area snugly with an elastic wrap, being careful not to cut off circulation. Wrap from below the injured area toward the heart. For a fracture, stabilize or immobilize on the ground or with a splint if movement is needed.
  - **C** = Apply a **cold** pack or crushed ice placed in a plastic bag to the injured area. Place a layer of gauze or cloth between the cold or ice pack and the skin to prevent damaging the skin. Leave the ice pack on for 20 to 30 minutes. If you do not have ice or a cold pack, soak the injured part in cold water or, in warmer months, wrap the part in wet cotton. DO NOT apply an ice or cold pack directly on an open fracture site.
  - **E** = **Elevate** the injured area above the heart level if possible. DO NOT elevate if you suspect a fracture or if moving the injured area causes pain.
- After 20 to 30 minutes of RICE, remove the cold and let the joint warm naturally for 10 to 15 minutes before testing to determine whether the joint can be used.
- The injury will heal faster if RICE is repeated 3 to 4 times a day until pain and swelling subside.

Splinting
Follow These Principles:

- In a wilderness or remote setting, chances are the patient will need to be moved. The general rule in the delayed-help situation is: "When in doubt, splint!"

- Splint only if you can do so without causing more pain.
- Remove rings, bracelets or watches from injured extremities.
- Make the splint out of something to pad the injury comfortably and something rigid enough to provide support.
- Fill in any hollows with soft padding.
- Be sure the splint is long enough to restrict the movement of the joints above and below a broken bone, or the movement of the bones above and below an injured joint.
- Prepare the splint before moving the limb.
- Splint an injury in the position of function or as close to it as possible. These positions include spine, neck and pelvis in-line, with padding in the small of the back (Figure 1); legs almost straight with padding behind the knees for slight flexion (Figure 2); feet at 90 degrees to legs (Figure 3); arms flexed to cross the heart (Figure 4); and hands in a functional curve with padding in the palms (Figure 5).
- Splint the injured area and the bones or joints above and below the injury.

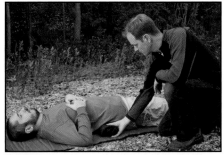

Figure 1

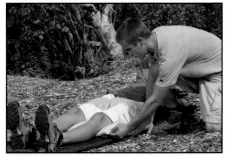

Figure 2

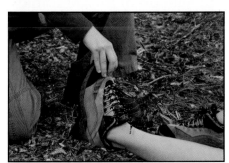

Figure 3

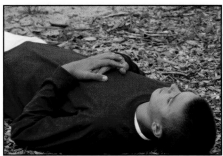

Figure 4

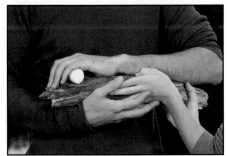

Figure 5

■ Attach the splint with a number of bandages tied securely with knots.

■ Monitor the injured area. Check CSM below the site of the injury before and after splinting and with every vital signs check. If there is no CSM, remove, loosen or reposition the splint.

Application of a Sling-and-Swathe (Sling and Binder)

■ Support the injured body part above and below the site of the injury.

■ Check for feeling, warmth and color.

■ Place a triangular bandage under the injured arm and over the uninjured shoulder to form a sling, keeping the wrist higher than the elbow.

■ Tie the ends of the sling at the side of the neck, placing padding beneath the knot.

■ Bind the injured body part to the chest with a folded triangular bandage.

■ Recheck for feeling, warmth and color (Figure 6).

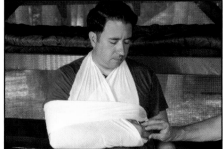

Figure 6

Application of an Anatomic Splint

■ Support the injured body part above and below the site of the injury.

■ Check for feeling, warmth and color.

■ For arms or legs, place several folded triangular bandages above and below the injured body part.

■ Place the uninjured body part next to the injured body part.

■ Tie triangular bandages securely. For fingers or toes, secure fingers to fingers and toes to toes with tape.

■ Recheck for feeling, warmth and color (Figure 7).

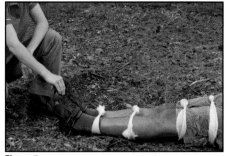

Figure 7

NOTE   If you are not able to check warmth and color because a sock or shoe is in place, check for sensation.

Application of a Soft Splint

- Support the injured body part above and below the site of the injury.
- Check for feeling, warmth and color.
- Place several folded triangular bandages above and below the injured body part.
- Gently wrap a soft object (e.g., a folded blanket or pillow) around the injured body part.
- Tie triangular bandages securely with knots.
- Recheck for feeling, warmth and color (Figure 8).

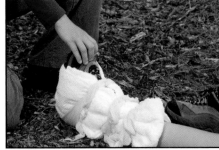

Figure 8

NOTE   If you are not able to check warmth and color because a sock or shoe is in place, check for sensation.

Application of a Rigid Splint

- Support the injured body part above and below the site of the injury.
- Check for feeling, warmth and color.
- Place the rigid splint (e.g., a board) under the injured body part and the joints that are above and below the injured body part.
- Tie several folded triangular bandages above and below the injured body part.
- Recheck for feeling, warmth and color (Figure 9).

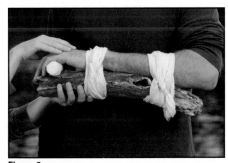

Figure 9

NOTE   If a rigid splint is used on an injured forearm, immobilize the wrist and elbow. Bind the arm to the chest using folded triangular bandages or apply a sling.

Strains and Sprains

⊘ When CHECKing the patient:

- Have the patient actively move the injured joint and evaluate the pain involved.
- Move the joint yourself and evaluate the patient's response.
- If the joint appears to be usable, have the patient test it with his or her body weight.
- Tell the patient not to use the injured part if movement causes pain.
- If the injury is to the lower part of the body and the patient can use the injured part without pain, offer to provide an appropriate support (e.g., for an injured knee, provide a walking splint, which restricts movement of the knee without putting pressure on the kneecap).

⊚ To give CARE:

- Splint any injured bone or joint that the patient cannot use.

Fractures

⊘ When CHECKing the patient:

- Determine if the injured part looks broken by comparing it to the uninjured side. Ask the patient if he or she thinks the part is broken.
- Gently touch the injured area and look for these signs of a fracture:
  - The patient reacts to your touch.
  - The muscles appear to be spasming.
  - The injured area feels unstable.
  - One spot hurts noticeably more than others.
- Check for CSM beyond the site of the injury. Loss of a pulse, numbness, tingling and inability to move are all signs of serious fracture-related complications.

⊚ To give CARE:

General:

- Splint any injury that you suspect is a fracture.
- Continue to check CSM after splinting to ensure that circulation is not cut off.

For a jaw fracture:

- Hold the jaw in place with a wide wrap that goes around the head.
- Make sure the wrap can be removed quickly if the patient needs to vomit.

For a collarbone fracture:

- Secure with a sling-and-swathe.
- Make the sling from triangular bandages or improvise by lifting the tail of the patient's shirt up over the arm on the injured side and pinning it in place.
- Be sure the sling lifts the elbow to take pressure off the shoulder.

For a lower arm fracture (including the wrist and hand):

- Secure the injured part to a well-padded, rigid support and place it in a sling-and-swathe.
- Place a roll of something soft in the hand to keep it in a position of function. If bones of the hand are damaged, be sure to secure the hand to the splint with lots of padding.

For a broken finger:

- Tape the broken finger to nearby uninjured fingers with padding between the fingers.

For an upper arm fracture:

- Place the arm in a sling-and-swathe.
- Secure the broken bone to the patient's chest with a wide, soft wrap.

For a rib fracture:

- Protect the injured rib by supporting the arm on the injured side with a sling-and-swathe.
- DO NOT wrap a band snugly around the patient's chest.
- Encourage the patient to take deep breaths regularly, even if it hurts, to keep the lungs clear.
- Watch the patient for increasing trouble breathing.

For a pelvis or hip fracture:

■ Secure the patient on a rigid litter (stretcher) before attempting a carry-out.

■ Place wide conforming wraps (e.g., a sheet or blanket) and tie around the pelvis to provide some support and security.

■ Secure the legs comfortably to each other (Figure 10).

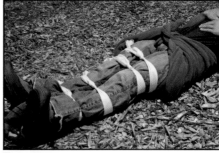
Figure 10

■ Be sure to watch the patient for signs and symptoms of shock due to internal bleeding, which is common with pelvic fractures.

For a leg fracture (including ankle and foot):

■ Secure the injured part on a well-padded, rigid support that includes immobilization of the ankle and foot.

■ Pad behind the knee for comfort.

Complicated Fractures

To give CARE:

For an angulated fracture:

If the limb is severely deformed or distorted, the bones may be straightened through gentle *in-line traction* to reduce pain. To do this:

■ Pull with gentle traction along the line in which the bone lies. This will relax the muscle and reduce the pain.

■ Slowly and gently move the broken bone back into normal alignment.

■ DO NOT use force.

■ DO NOT continue if the patient complains of increasing pain.

■ Splint the injury once the injured part is aligned.

For an open fracture:

■ Irrigate the wound and dress it appropriately. (Go to "Wounds" section for information on how to irrigate and dress the fracture.)

■ If bone ends stick out of the wound and a health care provider is longer than 4 to 6 hours away:

● Clean the wound and bone ends without touching them.

- Apply gentle in-line traction to the fracture to pull the bone ends back under the skin.
- Dress the wound.
- Splint the fracture.

Dislocations

Follow These Principles:

- The only treatment available for certain dislocations that occur in the wilderness is splinting in the most comfortable position.
- In other cases, the joint can be put back in its normal position through a process called *reduction.* If you are going to attempt a reduction, it is important that you:
    - Work quickly but calmly. Usually, the sooner a reduction is done, the easier it is on the injured patient and the responder.
    - Encourage the patient to relax, with particular concentration on the injured joint.
    - Stop if the pain increases dramatically.
    - Splint the injury after the joint is back in its normal position.

When **CHECK**ing the patient, look, listen and feel for:

- A joint that does not look "right." (Shoulder dislocations are the most common type.)
- Pain and/or loss of normal range of motion.
- A bump, ridge or hollow that does not normally exist.

To give **CARE**:

For a shoulder dislocation:

- Use the *Stimson technique* right away:
    - Position the patient face-down across a firm surface (e.g., a rock or log) with the arm on the injured side dangling down vertically.
    - Help the patient to relax.
    - With a soft cloth, tie something that weighs about 5 to 10 pounds to the dangling wrist.
    - Wait. This process takes about 20 to 30 minutes to work (Figure 11).

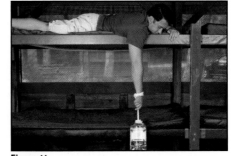

Figure 11

OR

- Have the injured patient perform a similar technique on him- or herself right away:
  - Standing or sitting, the patient should pull the injured arm straight and forward, away from the body, by gripping the wrist with the opposite hand (Figure 12).

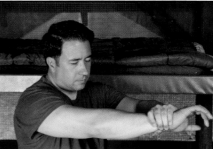

Figure 12

- Place the injured patient in a sling-and-swathe as soon as the shoulder is returned to its normal position.
- DO NOT bind the patient's arm in case he or she needs to use the arm in an emergency (e.g., escaping from an overturned raft).

For a finger or toe dislocation:

- Keeping the injured finger or toe partially flexed (bent), pull on the end with one hand while gently pressing the dislocated joint back into place with your other thumb (Figure 13).
- Place a gauze pad between the injured finger or toe and an uninjured neighboring finger or toe.

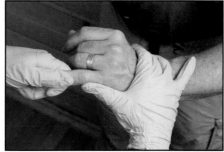

Figure 13

- Tape the injured finger or toe to the uninjured neighboring finger or toe.
- DO NOT tape directly over the joint itself.

For a kneecap dislocation:

- Apply gentle traction to the leg to straighten it out. This may cause the kneecap to pop back into place without any further treatment.
- If the kneecap does not pop back into place after the leg is straightened, massage the thigh and use your hand to push the kneecap gently back into normal alignment.
- Apply a splint that does not put pressure on the kneecap. This way, the patient may be able to walk.

◉ CALLing for Help: Guidelines for Evacuation

- If a patient is able to use the injured body part, the patient's degree of discomfort should determine whether and how to evacuate.
- Evacuate slowly–**GO SLOW**–anyone who cannot use the injured body part or who is suffering from a first-time dislocation. You might be able to avoid evacuation if the injury is to the outer joints of the fingers or toes.
- Evacuate rapidly–**GO FAST**–anyone with an angulated fracture; open fracture; fracture of the pelvis, hip or thigh; or more than one long bone fracture.
- Evacuate rapidly–**GO FAST**–anyone whose injuries create a decrease in CSM beyond the injury itself.

Burns

Burns are caused by heat, chemical reactions, electricity (including lightning) and radiation (including sunburn). The severity of a burn is determined by its depth (superficial, partial-thickness or full-thickness) and its extent (how much of the body's surface it covers).

⊘ When **CHECK**ing the patient, determine the depth of the burn:

- Superficial burns (Figure 1, A and B)
  - Red, painful and possibly swollen skin

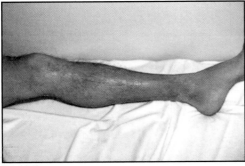

Figure 1A

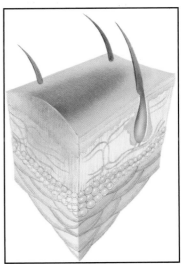

Figure 1B

- Partial-thickness burns (Figure 2, A and B)
  - Red, painful and swollen skin
  - Blisters, which sometimes form more than an hour after cooling

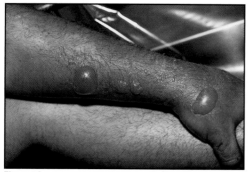

Figure 2A

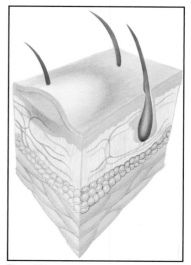

Figure 2B

- Full-thickness burns (Figure 3, A and B)
  - Painless skin without blisters
  - Pale skin (if injured by scalding)
  - Charred skin (if injured by fire)

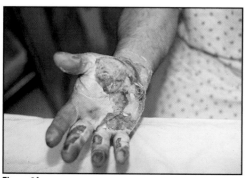

Figure 3A

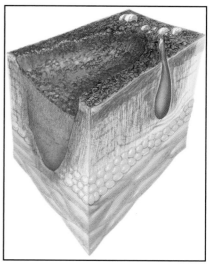

Figure 3B

When CHECKing the patient, determine the extent of the burn:

- Percentage of total body surface area (TBSA) that is burned
  - Use the Rule of Palmar Surface: The patient's palmar surface (inner surface of palm and fingers) equals 1 percent of TBSA.
  - The more TBSA that is burned, the more serious the injury.

NOTE   ■ Suspect possible airway complications with:
- Burns to the face and/or neck (Figure 4).
- Soot in the mouth and/or nose.
- Singed facial hair.
- A dry cough.

■ Major electrical burns (e.g., those caused by lightning or electrocution) may affect cardiac or respiratory systems. Always care for cardiac and respiratory problems before caring for burns.

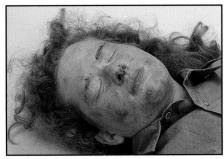
Figure 4

⊘ To give CARE:

■ Remove the patient from the source of the burn and immediate danger.

■ Stop the burning process quickly, within 30 seconds if possible.
- Remove the heat source.
- Smother flames.
- DO NOT try to remove tar, melted plastic or other material stuck to the burn.
- If electrical, turn off electricity FIRST.
- If dry chemical, brush off the chemical or remove contaminated clothing, then flood with water. Take precautions from breathing in dust. Make sure the chemical is not flushed onto other parts of the body.

■ Cool or flood the burn with cold water for at least 20 minutes (Figure 5).

■ Gently wash a mild burn with soap and water and pat dry.

■ Leave burn blisters intact.

■ Remove jewelry from burned area, if possible, to prevent complications resulting from swelling.

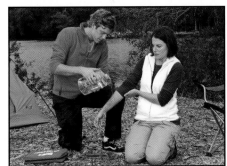
Figure 5

■ Dress the burn with a thin layer of antibiotic ointment.
- If ointment or dressings are not available, leave the burn alone. The burn's surface will dry into a scab-like covering that provides a significant amount of protection.

- Cover the burn with a gauze pad or a thin layer of roll gauze or apply clean clothing (Figure 6).
- DO NOT pack burn wounds or the patient in ice.
- Elevate burned extremities to minimize swelling.
- Have the patient gently and regularly move burned areas as much as possible.

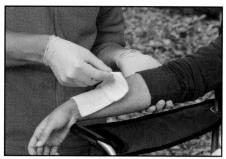

Figure 6

- Manage ABCDEs and protect the patient from shock and hypothermia.
- Keep the patient well hydrated and monitor burns as you would any open wound.
- Re-dress the injury twice a day by:
  - Removing old dressings by soaking off with clean, tepid water if needed.
  - Rewashing the wound to remove the old ointment.
  - Applying a clean covering.
- Re-dressing or re-examining a burn for infection is most likely going to be very painful. If evacuation is imminent (within hours to a day)—do not re-dress the burn.

CALLing for Help: Guidelines for Evacuation

- Evacuate rapidly—**GO FAST**—anyone with:
  - Trouble breathing.
  - A partial- or full-thickness burn that covers 10 percent or more of the patient's TBSA.
  - A partial- or full-thickness burn that is circumferential (wrapping around the body part), covering the entire hand, foot or other body part.
  - Serious burns of the head, face, neck, hands, feet or genitals.
  - A full-thickness burn that covers more than 5 percent of the TBSA.
  - Burns caused by chemicals, explosions or electricity.
  - Any partial- or full-thickness burn to a child or an elderly patient (younger than about age 5 or older than about age 60).

Chest Injuries

Any significant injury to the chest may lead to difficulty breathing, a potentially serious and life-threatening problem.

Chest Injuries (General)

⊘ When **CHECK**ing the patient, look, listen and feel for:

- Deformity, open injuries, tenderness and swelling (DOTS).
- Windpipe/trachea pushed to one side of the neck.
- Abnormal breathing (posture, rate, quality).
- After exposing the chest and back:
  - Bleeding or holes, with or without bubbles, and bruising.
  - Unusual noises like gurgling.
  - Abnormal chest rise.
- Guarding of the injury (patient is protecting it from being moved or touched).
- While exerting some pressure with your hands:
  - Cracking or crumbling sounds or depressions.
  - Pain or point tenderness along the ribs or clavicle.

Rib Injuries

⊘ When **CHECK**ing the patient, look, listen and feel for:

- Pain in the rib or clavicle area.
- Pain that increases when a deep breath is taken.
- Discoloration (bruising) where a rib may be broken and/or swelling.
- Guarding of the injury (patient is protecting it from being moved or touched).
- A point where the injury is most intense when touched.

♡ To give **CARE**:

- For a simple fractured rib, apply a sling-and-swathe to help ease discomfort and protect the area.
- DO NOT wrap a band snugly around the patient's chest.

- Encourage the patient to regularly take deep breaths, even if it hurts, to keep the lungs clear of fluid, particularly if an evacuation will be lengthy.
- Be aware of increasing trouble breathing.
- Offer the patient a bulky jacket or pillow to hold against his or her side for added comfort (Figure 1).

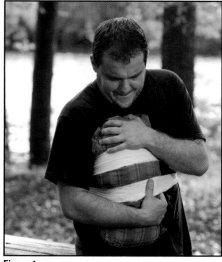

Figure 1

Lung Injuries

When **CHECK**ing the patient, look, listen and feel for:

- Presence of a *pneumothorax* (air escaping the lung and collecting in the chest). Signs and symptoms include:
  - Increased trouble breathing.
  - Rising level of anxiety.
- Presence of a *tension pneumothorax*. Signs and symptoms include:
  - Inability to breathe adequately, which can lead to death.

  NOTE   Evacuate the patient rapidly–**GO FAST**–as these are life-threatening conditions.

Flail Chest

⊘ When **CHECK**ing the patient, look, listen and feel for:

- A segment of ribs broken in two or more places; this part of the chest wall will move opposite of the rest of the chest (Figure 2, A and B).

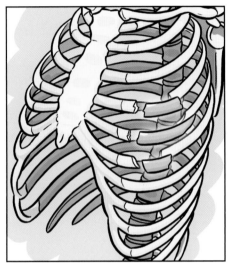

Figure 2A

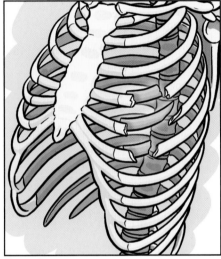

Figure 2B

◉ To give **CARE**:

- Tape a bulky dressing over the flail to allow the patient to breathe more easily.
  - DO NOT tape around the entire chest. This makes breathing more difficult.

  NOTE Evacuate the patient rapidly–**GO FAST**–as this is a life-threatening condition.

Sucking Chest Wound

⊘ When **CHECK**ing the patient, look, listen and feel for:

- Bubbling and noises coming from the wound when the patient breathes.

◉ To give **CARE**:

- Immediately cover the hole with an *occlusive dressing* that does not let air or water pass through. Clear plastic will work.

- Tape the dressing down securely on three sides (Figure 3).
- If the patient has difficulty breathing, remove the dressing. A tension pneumothorax could be developing. Removing the plastic may allow air in the chest to be released (Figure 4).
- If removing the dressing does not help breathing, consider gently pushing a gloved finger into the hole to release trapped air.
- If an object is sticking out of the chest, stabilize and pack it. DO NOT remove the object.

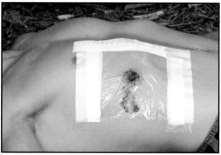

Figure 3

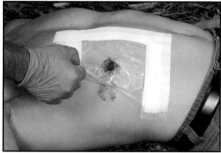

Figure 4

CALLing for Help: Guidelines for Evacuation

- Evacuate rapidly—**GO FAST**—anyone with a pneumothorax or tension pneumothorax. These are life-threatening injuries. There is no wilderness first aid treatment available other than care for a fractured rib.
- Evacuate rapidly—**GO FAST**—anyone who has sustained a chest injury associated with increased trouble breathing.
  - In this circumstance, the patient will need to be transported.
- Evacuate rapidly—**GO FAST**—anyone with a flail chest. This is a life-threatening injury.
  - Evacuate anyone with flail chest on his or her side with the injured side down or in another position of comfort.
  - Give rescue breaths during evacuation, if necessary.
- Evacuate slowly—**GO SLOW**—anyone with a suspected fractured rib.
  - Often, a patient with this injury is able to walk. A simple fractured rib must be evaluated by a health care provider.
  - Be sure to watch the patient for increased breathing difficulty. If this happens—**GO FAST**.

Head (Brain), Neck and Spinal Injuries

A significant blow to the head can cause bleeding and swelling of the brain. The skull is not large enough to handle much swelling, so brain injuries can cause death relatively quickly.

Superficial Scalp Injuries

⊘ When **CHECK**ing the patient, look, listen and feel for:
- Bleeding, which may be heavy at times.
- A bump on the head.

♡ To give **CARE**:
- Care for wounds as appropriate.
  - For a bleeding scalp, apply light (diffuse) pressure from a bulky dressing on the bleeding scalp. DO NOT apply direct pressure (Figure 1).
  - For a bump, apply a cold pack to reduce swelling.

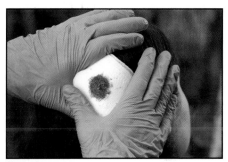

Figure 1

Mild Brain Injuries

⊘ When **CHECK**ing the patient, look, listen and feel for:
- Short-term (less than 3 minutes) or no loss of consciousness.
- Short-term amnesia (memory loss).
- Briefly blurred vision.
- Nausea.
- Headache.
- Dizziness.
- Lethargy (extreme tiredness and sluggishness).
- Possible neck pain or tenderness (if associated with spinal injury).

To give **CARE**:

- Care for wounds as appropriate.
  - Apply pressure from a bulky dressing on the bleeding scalp.
  - Apply a cold pack to a bump.
- Monitor the patient for 24 hours.
- Awaken the patient every 2 hours to check for signs and symptoms of serious brain damage.

Serious Brain Injuries

When **CHECK**ing the patient, look, listen and feel for:

- Prolonged unconsciousness with no response to aggressive stimulation, such as shouting or tapping the shoulder.
- Possible skull fracture. Signs and symptoms of a skull fracture include:
  - A depression (pressed-in area) in the skull. (DO NOT push on the area.)
  - A fracture that is visible where the scalp has been torn.
  - Bruising around both eyes (raccoon eyes) (Figure 2) or behind both ears (Figure 3).
  - Clear fluid and/or blood dripping from the nose or ears.
- Inability to sense touch or move extremities.
- Eyes that do not respond to light appropriately or equally. (Check pupil response, one eye at a time, by shading the eyes with a hand and then exposing the pupils to light.)
- Mental status deterioration (from disorientation, to irritability, to combativeness, to coma).
- Personality changes.
- Loss of coordination, balance and/or speech.
- Extremely bad headaches.

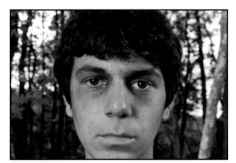

Figure 2

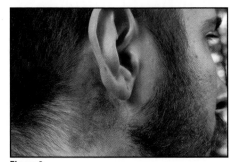

Figure 3

- Vision problems.
- Seizures.
- Nausea and vomiting that does not go away.
- Relapsing into unconsciousness.

In later stages:

- Heart rate that slows down (less than 40 beats per minute [BPM]), then speeds up.
- Erratic (irregular) respiratory rate.
- Unequal pupils.

> **NOTE** Without an obvious skull fracture, the patient may at first appear to have recovered, but later may start to deteriorate. Watch for signs and symptoms of brain injury whether or not you find evidence of a skull fracture.

To give **CARE**:

- Immobilize the patient and assume he or she may also have a spinal injury. See Spinal Injuries.
- Keep the patient calm and reassured.

> **NOTE** Evacuate the patient rapidly–**GO FAST**–as this could become a life-threatening condition.

CALLing for Help: Guidelines for Evacuation

- Evacuate anyone who sustained a blow to the head and does not respond initially to aggressive arousal attempts.
- If the patient is responsive and there is no indication of serious head or neck injury, he or she can walk out.
  - Make sure the patient is able to walk by testing his or her balance. Ask the patient to stand still with eyes closed. Swaying and/or falling may indicate brain injury.
  - Make sure the terrain is safe. If the terrain does not allow a second person to assist directly, DO NOT allow a patient with questionable balance to walk out.
- Evacuate rapidly–**GO FAST**–anyone with signs and symptoms of severe head (brain) injury, especially a skull fracture or stroke, and/or a decrease in mental status.
- Patients with serious head injuries should be carried.

- If the patient is unconscious, the airway must remain open during evacuation.
  - Keep the airway open by keeping the patient in a stable side position (the high arm in endangered spine [H.A.IN.E.S.] position).
  - Alternatively, if a patient has been placed on a rigid backboard for a

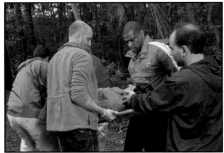

Figure 4

spinal injury, elevate the head end of the board approximately 6 to 8 inches (Figure 4). See Spinal Injuries.

Spinal Injuries

Damage to the spinal cord can cause permanent paralysis or death. Any possible spinal injury warrants evacuation, and due to the severity of the situation you **must** seek professional evacuation by an organized rescue party.

Mechanism of Injury

Suspect a spinal injury if the mechanism of injury (MOI) involves any of the following:

- Falling from a height or landing on the head or spine
- Falls on the buttocks that transmit force to the spine
- Any fall of a distance greater than the person's height
- Having the chin forced to the chest
- Excessive extension or rotation, such as tumbling downhill without skis releasing
- Pulling/jerking of the head from the neck
- Gunshot, stabbing or other injury that penetrates the body in the area of the spine
- Sudden and violent deceleration (decrease in speed)
- Any injury that causes a helmet to break
- Any diving mishap
- A motor vehicle crash involving a driver or passengers not wearing safety belts
- Being thrown from a motor vehicle or by an animal
- A lightning strike

A person found unconscious for unknown reasons should be considered spine injured.

✅ When **CHECK**ing the patient, look, listen and feel for:

- Spinal pain or tenderness to the touch.
- Obvious injury to the spinal column.
- Altered sensations in the extremities, such as numbness, tingling, unusual weakness, inability to move or unusual hot or cold sensations.
- Respiratory difficulty.
- Loss of bowel control.
- Signs and symptoms of shock.

💙 To give **CARE**:

- During the primary assessment, keep the patient's head still by placing hands on both sides of the patient's head, gently holding and supporting the head in the position in which it was found (*manual stabilization*) (Figure 5).

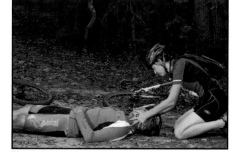

Figure 5

- Manage ABCDEs.
  - Use a modified jaw thrust to open or maintain airway if trained and if needed.
  - If you must remove a helmet, keep the patient's head still while removing the helmet. Remove a helmet only if:
    - The face mask cannot be removed reasonably quickly to gain access to the airway.
    - The design of the helmet and chin strap, even in the absence of the face mask, does not allow for an open airway or adequate breathing.
    - The design of the helmet and chin straps does not hold the head securely in place (immobilization of the helmet does not also immobilize the head).
    - The helmet prevents immobilization of the patient for transport in an appropriate position.
- Prevent further injury by immobilizing the head, neck and back.
- Check circulation, sensation and motion (CSM) before and after any movement of the patient.

- If the patient's head lies at an odd angle, straighten it with slow, gentle movement to line it up with the rest of the spine. This improves the airway and makes immobilization easier.
  - If this movement causes pain or meets resistance, stop and immobilize the patient's head as it lies.
- If the patient is found crumpled into an odd body position, straighten the body with slow, gentle movement of one body part at a time. This typically makes the patient more comfortable and provides for better immobilization.
- Once the spine is in alignment, apply a cervical collar to restrict motion.

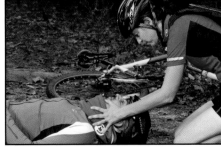

Figure 6

  - Use a commercial collar, if available, or improvise one using such items as rolled clothing, a piece of a foam sleeping pad or rolled towels (Figure 6).
  - Make sure the collar goes completely around the patient's neck. If the improvised collar varies in thickness, place the thickest part between the chin and chest.
  - Be careful not to exert pressure on the trachea (windpipe).
- Maintain in-line stabilization, if possible, while you wait for a rigid litter (stretcher) to arrive for evacuation. If not possible, place barriers on either side of head to prevent movement (e.g., sand bags, large water containers).
- When a litter arrives, make sure the patient is made free of any movement (FOAM) on the litter.
  - Use pads to fill any spaces under the knees, in the small of the back and any other space that would allow the patient to shift.
  - Strap the patient's head down last (Figure 7).
- Repeat hands-on physical exam periodically. Observe and record for at least 24 hours.

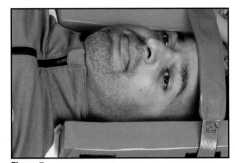

Figure 7

Moving a Patient with a Head or Spinal Injury
Log Roll (To check for injury)

A log roll can be used to roll a patient with a suspected spinal injury onto his or her side to check the back for injuries. It can also be used to place a pad underneath the patient. Although it is possible for one responder to perform a log roll, two or three responders make the job easier and safer for the patient.

To give CARE:

- Have one responder position him- or herself at the injured patient's head and perform manual stabilization.
- At the command of that responder, roll the patient as a unit, keeping the neck and back in line (Figure 8).
- Hold the patient stable while the back is checked for injuries.
- Roll the patient back using the same precautions.

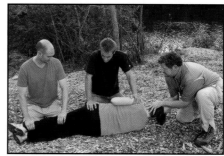
Figure 8

> NOTE The log roll can be used to move an injured patient from side to back and from face-down to back.

BEAM (To move a short distance)

The body elevation and movement (BEAM) technique can be used to move a patient with a possible spinal injury a short distance when there are other responders available to help.

To give CARE:

- Designate and prepare the spot to which the patient will be carried.
- Have one responder position him- or herself at the patient's head and perform manual stabilization.
- Have the other responders kneel on both sides of the patient. These responders gently slide their hands under the patient.
- At the command of the head-holder, the group lifts the patient as a unit with as little spinal movement as possible.
- The group carries the patient to the designated spot and then, at the command of the head-holder, lowers the patient.

Cautions About Moving a Spine-Injured Patient

- The only reasons to move a spine-injured patient in a safe scene are to improve long-term comfort, give essential care and/or to protect the patient from the environment.
- The least amount of movement is best. More harm can be done during improper transfer than through any other action associated with first aid.
- Transfer of a patient should be done only when absolutely necessary or when the risk for further injury is low.
- Always make sure the airway is open and serious bleeding has been stopped.
- Before moving the patient, make sure initial pain and fear have subsided and be sure to reassure the patient.
- Plan ahead so that the patient is moved only once.
- Prepare any insulating materials or shelter before the patient is moved.
- Rehearse and practice the process before moving the patient.
- The rescuer supporting the head is the leader and should act and be treated as such.
- Protection of the patient's entire body must be assured during the move. The body should be kept in a straight line.

Special Considerations: Focused Spine Assessment

If the MOI caused you to suspect a spinal injury but a full assessment did not reveal any signs and symptoms, perform a focused spine assessment. If you answer "yes" to all of these questions, discontinue spinal immobilization:

- Is the patient fully reliable (assessed on the AVPU scale as at least A+O×3)? Does he or she appear sober and without distractions, such as severely painful injuries or deep psychological distress?
- Is the patient without altered sensations in the extremities, such as tingling, and does he or she have the ability to move the extremities?
- Does the patient demonstrate grip strength and the ability to lift the legs against resistance?
- Does the patient deny feeling spinal pain and tenderness to the touch of the spine, and does he or she have normal range of motion?

◎ CALLing for Help: Guidelines for Evacuation

- Possible spinal injury is a serious condition. Always seek professional evacuation by an organized rescue party.
- Evacuate rapidly–**GO FAST**–anyone with the signs and symptoms of spinal cord injury.

Heat-Related Illnesses

Heat Exhaustion

Heat exhaustion is a result of a combination of factors that may include heat stress, water and electrolyte loss (most often via sweat), and inadequate hydration, usually by a person who has been exercising.

⊘ When **CHECK**ing the patient, look, listen and feel for:

- Sweating.
- Exhaustion.
- Pale, sweaty or flushed skin.
- Headache.
- Nausea and/or vomiting.
- Muscle cramps.
- Thirst and decreased urine output (urine is yellowish).
- Dizziness when the person stands up quickly.
- Elevated heart rate and respiratory rate.
- Slightly elevated core temperature (not common).

♡ To give **CARE**:

- Have the patient stop activity and rest, preferably in a cool, shady place.
- Help the patient replace lost fluids and salt.
  - Give him or her water with a pinch of table salt, water with oral rehydration salts, water along with a salty snack or a diluted sports drink.
- DO NOT give salt tablets, as they are too concentrated.
- Wet down and fan the patient to increase the rate of cooling.
- Gently massage and stretch cramped muscles.
- If drowsy, allow the patient to sleep.
- Allow the patient to continue with normal activity if he or she feels better.
- Recovery may take up to 24 hours. Continue to observe the patient for recurrences.

Heat Stroke

Heat stroke is a serious medical emergency. It often occurs when a person is over-exerting him- or herself and/or seriously dehydrated. The body produces heat faster than it can be shed.

⊘ When CHECKing the patient, look, listen and feel for:

- Core temperature of 105° F (104° F oral temperature) or more.
- Disorientation and bizarre personality changes.
- Hot, red and sometimes dry skin.
- Elevated heart rate and respiratory rate.
- Headache.
- Seizures.

♡ To give CARE:

- Rapid cooling is the only way to save the patient.
- Move the patient to a cooler environment.
- Remove heat-retaining clothing and immerse the patient in cold water until he or she becomes alert (Figure 1).

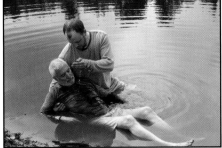

Figure 1

- If a large enough source of water is not available for immersion, drench the patient with cold water.
  - Concentrate on the head and the neck.
  - Use cold packs on the neck, armpits, groin, hands and feet.
  - Fan the patient constantly to increase evaporation.
- Monitor the patient closely and stop cooling efforts when a normal mental status returns.
- Give cold water if the patient is able to accept and drink it.
- DO NOT give fever-reducing drugs.
- The patient must see a health care provider as soon as possible, even if he or she appears to have recovered.
- Carefully watch the patient during evacuation. Relapses are common.

Hyponatremia

Hyponatremia is a condition that occurs when the sodium level in a person's blood falls too low to maintain normal body function. It is usually the result of drinking too much water and failing to eat. If untreated, hyponatremia will result in seizures, coma and death.

⊘ When CHECKing the patient, look, listen and feel for:

- Headache.
- Weakness and fatigue.
- Light-headedness.
- Muscle cramps.
- Nausea, with or without vomiting.
- Sweaty skin.
- Clear urine; person has recently urinated.
- Person recently drank a lot of water.
- Normal core or oral temperature.
- Normal or slightly elevated pulse and breathing.
- Increasing level of anxiety.
- Altered mental status including disorientation, irritability and combativeness (in severe cases, this is referred to as water intoxication).

♡ To give CARE:

- Have the patient rest in shade with no fluid intake and a gradual intake of salty foods while the kidneys re-establish a sodium balance.
- Once a patient develops hunger and thirst combined with normal urine output, the condition has resolved. Evacuation is not necessary unless the patient has an altered mental status.

NOTE
- A patient with hyponatremia will appear to have heat exhaustion. DO NOT treat it as heat exhaustion (i.e., give water). This will harm the person.
- Use these guidelines to distinguish between heat exhaustion and hyponatremia:
  - Persons with heat exhaustion typically have a low output of yellowish urine (urinating every 6 to 8 hours) and are thirsty.
  - Hyponatremic persons have urinated recently and the urine was probably clear.
  - Hyponatremic persons will also claim to have been drinking a lot of water and/or deny being thirsty.

CALLing for Help: Guidelines for Evacuation

- Evacuate rapidly–**GO FAST**–anyone with an altered mental status or who has had a seizure as a result of heat stroke.
- Evacuate slowly–**GO SLOW**–anyone who does not fully recover from heat exhaustion or mild hyponatremia.

Hypothermia

Hypothermia is the lowering of the body's core temperature to a point at which normal brain and/or muscle function is impaired. This condition can be mild, moderate or life threatening.

Mild to Moderate Hypothermia

When CHECKing the patient, look, listen and feel for:
With mild hypothermia:

- Shivering.
- The "umbles":
  - Inability to perform complex tasks ("fumbles").
  - Confusion, apathy and sluggish thinking ("grumbles").
  - Slurred speech ("mumbles").
  - Altered gait ("stumbles").
- The patient being able to eat and talk and usually complaining of feeling cold.

With moderate hypothermia:

- Worsening of the "umbles."
- Uncontrollable, violent shivering.
- Confusion or unusual behavior.
- Impaired judgment.

To give CARE:
For mild to moderate hypothermia:

- Change the environment to prevent heat loss.
  - Place the patient out of wind and cold and into some kind of shelter, even if this is only waterproof, windproof clothing.

- Cover all exposed skin, including the patient's head and neck.
- Replace wet clothes with something dry.
- If the patient can eat, give simple carbohydrates, such as candy and juice (Figure 1).
  - If the patient can drink, give fluids, preferably a warm, sweet drink (e.g., warm gelatin dessert). Give cold fluids if warm ones are not available.
  - DO NOT give the patient caffeine and/or alcohol.

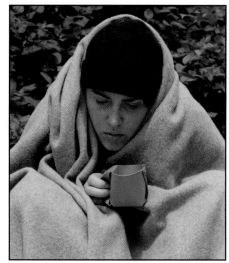

Figure 1

- If the patient cannot exercise muscles easily, try to keep him or her warm by:
  - Insulating him or her from the ground.
  - Bundling him or her in dry insulation.
  - Having him or her snuggle with warm people, such as in a sleeping bag. If the patient goes to sleep, wake him or her periodically.
  - Placing a hot water bottle or chemical heat packs near the heart and in the armpits and groin area (but not against bare skin).
- Wait until the patient returns to normal and is able to exercise muscles before you keep moving.
- If the patient can still exercise easily, you can continue activity after initial care.

Severe Hypothermia

When **CHECK**ing the patient, look, listen and feel for:

- Patient stops shivering.
- Increasing muscle rigidity.
- Worsening mental state, moving from stupor to coma.
- Decreasing pulse and breathing that become difficult to detect (but are still present).
- Semi-consciousness or unconsciousness.
- Patient stops complaining.
- A core temperature lower than 90° F.

⚕ To give **CARE**:

- Handle the patient with severe hypothermia gently—roughness can overload a cold heart and stop it.
- If breathing is undetectable, perform rescue breathing or cardiopulmonary resuscitation (CPR) for at least 3 minutes prior to any movement.
- Take steps to get the patient warm (see mild to moderate hypothermia care steps).
- Create a "hypothermia wrap" vapor barrier to trap any heat still left in the patient.
  - Wrap the patient with a tent fly, sheet of plastic, garbage bags or other items available to trap any heat remaining in the patient (Figure 2, A and B).
  - The hypothermia wrap should resemble a cocoon in that it only opens to the mouth and nose.
- DO NOT try to force food or drink.
- Care for severe hypothermia even if the patient appears dead. DO NOT assume a patient is dead unless he or she has been re-warmed and is not responding to any care given.
- Call for help immediately.
- Evacuate the patient gently. DO NOT evacuate if it cannot be done gently.

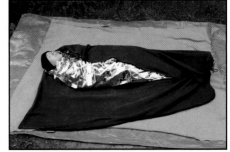

Figure 2A

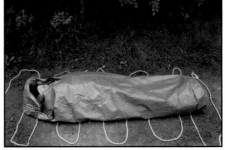

Figure 2B

> **NOTE** Warming the body too quickly or moving the patient too much will likely send the cold blood to the core, causing the body temperature to drop even further. This can be fatal because the heart does not function properly when it is cold.

◉ **CALL**ing for Help: Guidelines for Evacuation

- Anyone who has recovered from mild to moderate hypothermia may remain in the field.
- Evacuate rapidly—**GO FAST** but with extreme gentleness—anyone with severe hypothermia.

Lightning

Prevent Lightning Injuries

What to do (before a possible lightning storm arrives):

- Pick campsites that meet safety precautions.
- Know local weather patterns, especially in summertime.
  - Plan turnaround times (the amount of time you need to get back) in lightning-prone areas, based on your research, and stick to the plan.
- Plot storms using the following method:
  - When the flash of lightning precedes the boom of thunder by 5 seconds, the storm is approximately 1 mile away.
  - Follow the 30-30 rule: Seek a safe location when the storm is no less than 6 miles away. That is 30 seconds from flash to boom. Stay in the safe location for 30 minutes after the storm passes.

Reaching Safety in a Lightning Storm

What to do:

- Move downhill.
- Do not stay in a meadow or any other wide-open space.
- Seek uniform cover (e.g., low rolling hills or trees of about the same size).
- Take shelter in a steel-framed building or a hard-topped motor vehicle. Keep the windows of the vehicle rolled up.
- If you are boating or swimming, get to land and move away from the shore.
- AVOID all of the following:
  - Metal
  - Anything connected to electrical power
  - High places and high objects (e.g., tall trees)
  - Open places
  - Damp, shallow caves and tunnels
  - Overhangs
  - Flood zones
  - Places obviously struck by lightning in the past
  - Long conductors (e.g., fences)

- To assume a safe position
  when outdoors:
  - Squat or sit in a tight body position
    on insulating material (e.g., sleeping
    pad, life jacket) (Figure 1).
  - Take off any metal-framed packs
    and toss hiking poles away from
    the group.
  - DO NOT lie down.
  - If you feel your hair stand on end or your skin get tingly, cover your ears with your
    hands, close your eyes and get your head close to your knees.
- Spread groups out wide with about 100 feet or more between individuals.
  Keep everyone in sight if possible.

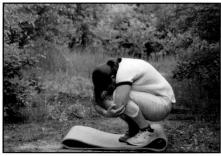

Figure 1

Lightning Injuries

Lightning can produce several types of injuries, including cardiac and pulmonary arrest, neurological problems, blindness, deafness, burns and trauma.

⊘ When **CHECK**ing the patient, look, listen and feel for:

- Burn marks on the skin (entry and exit of current).
- Unconsciousness.
- Trauma (e.g., fractures or dislocations).
- Dazed, confused behavior.
- Trouble breathing.
- Weak, irregular or absent pulse.

♡ To give **CARE**:

- Begin cardiopulmonary resuscitation (CPR) immediately if needed.
- Treat any injuries as needed.
- Be ready to treat secondary issues (e.g., hypothermia in a wet,
  injured person).

⦿ **CALL**ing for Help: Guidelines for Evacuation

- Evacuate rapidly—**GO FAST**—anyone who has been struck by lightning.
- Even if the patient seems to have recovered soon after the injury, serious
  problems can develop later so you must still evacuate rapidly.

Shock and Heart Attack

Shock

Shock is a condition that develops when the body's vital organs, including the brain, heart and lungs, do not get enough oxygen-rich blood to function properly. Shock is likely to develop after any serious injury or illness, including severe bleeding, severe allergic reaction, serious internal injury, significant fluid loss or dehydration, heart attack or other conditions. The goals of first aid are to get help quickly and give care to minimize shock while caring for the injury or illness.

⊘ When **CHECK**ing the patient, look, listen and feel for:

In the early stages of shock:

- Anxiousness, restlessness and/or disoriented level of responsiveness (LOR).
- Rapid and weak or otherwise irregular heart rate.
- Rapid and shallow respiratory (breathing) rate.
- Pale, cool, clammy skin color, temperature and moisture.
- Pink and warm skin color, temperature and moisture if shock was caused by an allergic reaction.
- Nausea and sometimes vomiting.
- Dizziness.
- Thirst.

In later stages of shock:

- LOR that continues to decrease.
- Eventual unresponsiveness.
- Heart rate in which the radial pulse (the pulse at the wrist) grows increasingly rapid, weakens and eventually disappears.

⊘ To give **CARE**:

- Identify and treat shock early, before serious signs and symptoms develop.
- Care for the condition that is causing the shock (e.g., bleeding, dehydration) immediately if it can be identified.
- Keep the patient calm and reassured.
- Have the patient lie down or move him or her into a position of comfort.
- Maintain an open airway.

- Give sips of cool water to prevent dehydration if the patient tolerates fluids and his or her mental status allows holding and drinking from a container.
- Elevate the patient's feet comfortably about 12 inches, unless injuries to the head or lower extremities prevent this.
- Keep the patient from getting chilled or overheated (e.g., use a sleeping pad to insulate the patient from the ground or cover the patient if shivering).
- DO NOT give fluids to an unconscious patient or to a patient with a serious head or abdominal injury.
- If the patient vomits, DO NOT give fluids. If evacuation will be delayed more than 1 hour, give small sips to drink every 5 minutes if tolerated without vomiting.

⊚ CALLing for Help: Guidelines for Evacuation

- If shock is not treated, it can lead to death. Options for care are limited in the wilderness, so early recognition and management are critical. Evacuation must be considered.
- Evacuate anyone with signs and symptoms of shock that do not stabilize or improve over time.
- Evacuate rapidly—**GO FAST**—anyone with decreased mental status or worsening vital signs, especially if the patient's heart rate keeps speeding up. The patient must be carried.

Heart Attack

Heart attack, due to an inadequate supply of oxygen-rich blood to the heart muscle, is the leading cause of death in the United States. A heart attack can, but does not always, lead to shock. Not only does shock make the situation more serious, it is usually fatal.

⊘ When CHECKing the patient, look, listen and feel for:

- Center-chest discomfort (e.g., crushing, squeezing pain, heavy pressure).
- Pain (e.g., crushing, squeezing pain, heavy pressure), mostly on the left side, which may radiate to the shoulder, down the arm or into the jaw.
- Nausea, sweating and shortness of breath.
- Denial of the possibility that this could be a heart attack.
- Unexplained fatigue.

To give **CARE**:

- Keep the patient physically and emotionally calm.
- DO NOT allow the patient to walk—even a short distance.
- Give the patient four 81-mg aspirins or one 325-mg aspirin, if the patient can swallow and has no known contraindications. Coated aspirin takes too long to dissolve to be effective, but can be taken if it is all you have on hand.
- If the patient has a strong radial pulse and has been prescribed nitroglycerin, help him or her self-administer one pill; it should be taken under the tongue with the patient sitting (Figure 1). Follow the instructions on the prescription.
- If the patient is unconscious and not breathing, immediately begin rescue breathing or cardiopulmonary resuscitation (CPR). If the patient does not have a pulse, immediately begin CPR or use an automated external defibrillator (AED), if one is available.

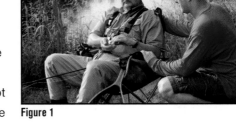

Figure 1

> **NOTE** The patient should only take medication if he or she can swallow and has no known contraindications. Patients should read and follow all label or health care provider instructions. Check state and local regulations regarding use of prescription and over-the-counter medications.

CALLing for Help: Guidelines for Evacuation

- Evacuate rapidly—**GO FAST**—anyone whom you assess as having a heart attack. The patient will need to be carried.

Submersion Incidents

The first step when dealing with any emergency is to determine that the scene is safe for the rescuer. A drowning person in the water can place a responder in a hazardous situation if the responder is unskilled in water rescue, particularly in an unsafe area. Fortunately, drowning can often be prevented with simple precautions, including the use of a safe area for swimming and matching activities to swimming ability. In murky water, where it would be difficult to find someone on the bottom, limit depths to shallow water or have all swimmers wear a life jacket. All boaters should wear a U.S. Coast Guard-approved personal flotation device (PFD) and be skilled with their craft in the local environment. It is important to gather rescue aids and discuss and practice rescue procedures before engaging in water activities.

You must first recognize that someone is in trouble and then choose a safe rescue procedure based on the behaviors you observe.

Helping a Person in Trouble in the Water

⊘ When **CHECK**ing the patient, look for these behaviors:

- Distressed swimmer (Figure 1)
  - Can breathe and might call for help
  - Can float, scull or tread water; might wave for help
  - Could be in horizontal, vertical or diagonal body position, depending on means of support
  - Makes little or no forward progress; less and less able to support self
  - May reach for rescue aids extended, thrown or pushed nearby

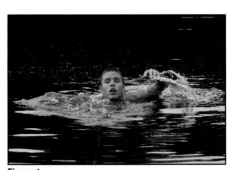

Figure 1

- Active drowning victim (Figure 2)
  - Struggles to breathe; cannot call out for help
  - Arms to sides alternately moving up and pressing down; no supporting kick
  - Vertical body position
  - No forward progress (has only 20 to 60 seconds before submerging)
  - Unable to reach for or move even a short distance to a rescue aid, but may be supported by an aid placed within his or her grasp
- Passive drowning victim (Figure 3)
  - Not breathing
  - No arm or leg action
  - Horizontal or vertical body position; could be face-down, face-up or submerged
  - No forward progress
  - Unable to grasp a rescue aid; assist normally requires contact by rescuer

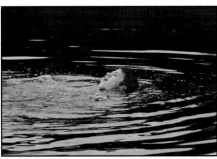

Figure 2

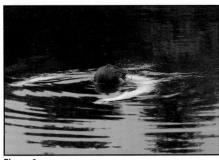

Figure 3

To assist the victim in the water:

- Continue to monitor the safety of everyone else (or have someone else do so) when attention is focused on an individual in trouble.
- Follow the progression of *Reach, Throw, Row, Go* based on your level of training. Out-of-water assists are safer for the responder. Ensure that you talk to the victim throughout the rescue to keep him or her calm and aware of your presence.
- If conditions are unsafe and beyond your level of training, stop your rescue efforts if the risk becomes unacceptable. For example, you should not attempt a rescue of a kayaker pinned in heavy white water unless you have specialized training in swift-water rescue.

■ Remember the progression of *Reach, Throw, Row, Go.*

1. *Reach* out to the person with a hand, foot, clothing, stick, paddle or anything that allows you to remain safely on land or in a boat (Figure 4).

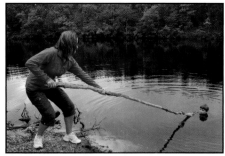

Figure 4

● Brace yourself on the pier surface, shoreline or another solid surface. Extend the object to the victim or reach with your arm and grasp the victim. When the victim grasps the object or when you grasp the victim, slowly and carefully pull him or her to safety. Keep your body low and lean back to avoid being pulled into the water.

● If you are in the water, hold on to a piling or another secure object with one hand. Extend your free hand or one of your legs to the victim. Do not let go of the secure object or swim out into the water. Pull the victim to safety.

● If the water is safe and shallow enough (not higher than your chest), you can wade in to reach the victim. Do not enter the water if there is a current, if the bottom is soft or if you do not know the condition of the bottom. If possible, wear a life jacket when attempting a wading assist, and take a buoyant object to extend your reach. Wade into the water and extend the object to the victim (Figure 5, A and B). When the victim grasps the object, tell him or her to hold on to the object tightly for support and pull him or her to safety. Keep the object between you and the victim to help prevent the victim from clutching at you in a panic.

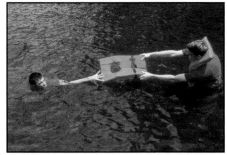

Figure 5A

2. *Throw* something that floats to the person so he or she can hold on to it. You can also throw a rope and tow the person to safety.

● Get into a stride position; the leg opposite your throwing arm is forward.

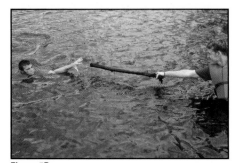

Figure 5B

- Step on the end of the line with your forward foot.
- Shout to get the victim's attention. Make eye contact and say that you are going to throw the object now. Tell the victim to grab it.
- Bend your knees and throw the object to the victim. Try to throw the object upwind and/or up current, just over the victim's head, so that the line drops within reach (Figure 6).
- When the victim has grasped the object or the line, slowly pull him or her to safety. Lean away from the water as you pull.
- If the object does not reach the victim, quickly pull the line back in and throw it again. Try to keep the line from tangling, but do not waste time trying to coil it. If using a throw bag, partially fill the bag with some water and throw it again.

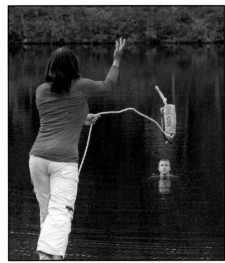

Figure 6

3. *Row* to the person, or get to the person in some sort of watercraft, using reaching or throwing devices as appropriate, with safety as a top priority (Figure 7).

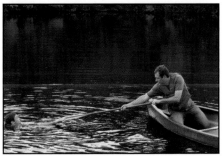

Figure 7

4. *Go.* "Go" is ONLY appropriate for good swimmers with water rescue training and when it is possible to safely reach the victim. The responder may wade or swim with a flotation aid toward a conscious victim, stop a safe distance away and then pass the flotation aid within the victim's grasp. Recovery of an unconscious victim may require a surface dive and contact tow. In murky water, limit water depth and/or require participants to wear life jackets to make underwater recovery easier if an incident occurs.

Caring for a Drowned Person (Once the person is removed from the water)

⊘ When **CHECK**ing the patient, look, listen and feel for:

- Unconsciousness.
- Airway.
- Breathing.
- Circulation.
- Disability.
- Environmental conditions.

♡ To give **CARE**:

- If the patient is not moving or breathing normally, begin rescue breathing or cardiopulmonary resuscitation (CPR).
- DO NOT attempt to clear the patient's lungs of water.
- Be ready to roll the patient to clear the airway if water or vomit comes up.
- If the patient has a suspected head, neck or back injury, take steps to immobilize the spine.

    NOTE Techniques for providing in-line stabilization for suspected head, neck and back injuries in the water for both face-up and face-down victims are covered in water rescue courses, such as American Red Cross Lifeguarding or Basic Water Rescue.

- Care for shock, hypothermia or other conditions as appropriate, including anything that might have caused the patient's distress in the water (e.g., diabetic emergency).

    NOTE Scuba diving introduces risks from breathing compressed air. Certified scuba divers are trained to avoid, recognize and arrange care for such problems. Care may require transport to a hyperbaric chamber.

📶 **CALL**ing for Help: Guidelines for Evacuation

- Evacuate rapidly–**GO FAST**–anyone who was unconscious, no matter how short a time, during a submersion incident. This situation can become life threatening.

- Evacuate rapidly—**GO FAST**—anyone with signs and symptoms of respiratory problems after a submersion incident or anyone who ingested water during a submersion incident. This situation can become life threatening. The patient should seek medical attention as soon as possible.

    NOTE   Secondary drowning is an aftereffect of water entering the lungs. It may take several days to appear. It can be fatal due to the water damage that occurs in the lungs.

Wounds and Wound Infection

Always follow standard precautions when dealing with bleeding to prevent the risk of disease transmission.

Bleeding

✅ When **CHECK**ing the patient, look, listen and feel for:

- Bleeding that spurts from the arteries each time the patient's heart beats. (This is life threatening.)
- Smooth and rapid bleeding from veins and at the surface. (This is also serious.)
- Signs of bruising. (This signals internal bleeding.)

✅ To give **CARE**:

- Look for serious bleeding with a quick visual scan (Figure 1).
- Check for bleeding inside clothing if the patient is wearing bulky winter or rain gear. Be sure to look for the site of the bleeding.
- Check for bleeding underneath the patient if he or she is lying in sand, rocks, snow or other terrain that could hide blood loss.

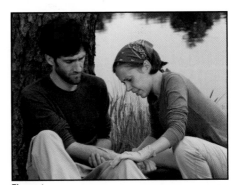

Figure 1

- Cover the wound with a sterile dressing and apply direct pressure to the bleeding wound with a barrier and your hand (Figure 2).
    - If there is no time to get a sterile dressing, grab anything absorbent to press into the wound.
    - If bleeding is severe, initially pack the wound with your fingers and then switch to packing with absorbent material.

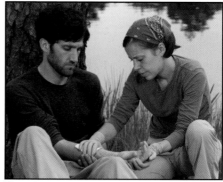

Figure 2

- DO NOT apply direct pressure to bleeding wounds of the head and neck.
    - **For neck wounds:** Carefully pinch the opening of the wound closed.
    - **For skull fractures:** Cover the wound with a bulky dressing and press lightly.
- Monitor the patient for shock.

Impaled Objects

⊕ To give CARE:

- DO NOT remove an object unless it interferes with urgent first aid (e.g., cardiopulmonary resuscitation [CPR]).
- Control severe bleeding by packing a bulky dressing around the object.
- Apply gentle pressure and immobilize the object by bandaging around it (Figure 3).
- Reduce the size and weight of the object if possible (e.g., by cutting off a tree limb).
- Remove a small impaled object in the skin (e.g., a splinter) with tweezers or similar tool.

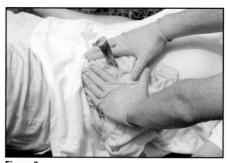

Figure 3

Tourniquets

Use a tourniquet on an arm or leg ONLY if blood loss is *uncontrolled* by direct pressure or if direct pressure is *not* possible. Situations might include:

- A disaster scene with multiple patients and limited rescuers.
- One patient with multiple injuries and one first aid provider.
- A patient who needs to be moved quickly or who is trapped without access to the wound.

⊚ To give **CARE**:

- Tie a band of soft material, about 4 inches wide, approximately 2 inches above the wound but not over the joint (Figure 4). DO NOT use anything narrow (e.g., rope or string).
- Tie a short, sturdy stick or another rigid object into the material and twist it (called the windlass technique) (Figure 5).
- Tighten the tourniquet by twisting until bleeding stops, and no more.
- In a non-delayed-help situation, continue to monitor and care for shock and keep the tourniquet tight and in place until the patient reaches advanced medical care (surgery will most likely be required).

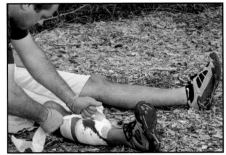

Figure 4

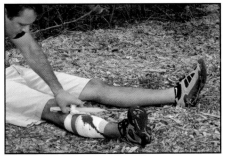

Figure 5

- Note the time that you applied the tourniquet.
- Tag the patient in an obvious place with information about when and where the tourniquet was placed.
- DO NOT cover the tourniquet with clothing.

Removing a Tourniquet

In a remote or wilderness situation, the goal is to release the tourniquet once the scene is safe and the patient is stable with direct pressure. Continuous use of a tourniquet will result in limb damage or loss.

⊚ To give CARE:

- If medical care is more than 2 hours away, you can release the tourniquet approximately every 2 hours to assess the continued need for the tourniquet.
  - Apply direct pressure to the wound.
  - Loosen the tourniquet, but leave it in place. Take 1 second to assess the bleeding.
  - If bleeding has remarkably slowed or stopped, substitute a pressure dressing for the tourniquet.
  - If bleeding remains persistent *with* direct pressure, replace the tourniquet.
  - DO NOT remove a tourniquet if there has been extensive blood loss, the patient is already in shock or you are unable to assess the amount of continued bleeding.

  NOTE   ■ Commercial emergency tourniquets are available and recommended. Follow manufacturer's instructions.

       ■ If a tourniquet is required for a lower leg wound and bleeding is not stopped when a tourniquet is placed near the wound, relocate the tourniquet to just above the knee. (This may work better because it is easier to compress the artery against the femur.)

       ■ It is better to continuously use a tourniquet than to allow additional blood loss.

Wound Cleaning

After bleeding is controlled, the wound should be properly cleaned, closed and dressed to prevent infection, promote healing and reduce scarring. This is often referred to as irrigating the wound.

⊚ To give CARE:

- Wash your hands.
- Put on clean, non-latex disposable gloves.
- Remove any large materials with tweezers or gauze pads before washing the wound.
- Vigorously wash and rinse dirty wounds with large amounts (at least 1 quart) of disinfected water or water that is potable (i.e., safe to drink). Disinfected water has been treated via boiling, chemicals or filtration—or some combination—to make it potable.

- Direct a high-pressure stream of water into the wound through an irrigation syringe, if available (Figure 6).
  - Draw the water into the syringe, hold the syringe about 2 inches above and perpendicular to the wound and push down forcefully on the plunger.

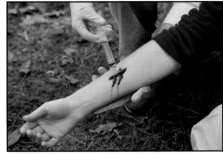

Figure 6

  - Keep the wound tipped so the water runs out.
- If no irrigation syringe is available, improvise by:
  - Using a biking water bottle.
  - Melting a pinhole in the center of the lid of a standard water bottle.
  - Punching a pinhole in a clean plastic bag.
- If the wound was initially washed using water that was not disinfected, follow up with a final flush of disinfected or potable water.
- DO NOT use hydrogen peroxide, rubbing alcohol or tincture of iodine, as these can further damage tissue.

NOTE
- Flaps of skin may need to be held open while the wound is being washed.
- Skin around a laceration should be washed clean before irrigating the wound.
- Puncture wounds need considerable irrigation because they are deep and have the potential for infection, especially with animal bites.

Wound Dressing and Closing

Lacerations

Lacerations are cuts through the skin that have even or ragged edges (Figure 7).

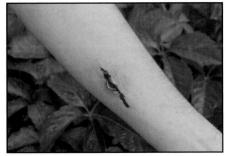

Figure 7

⊙ To give **CARE**:

■ If the wound is a laceration that you held open while cleaning, close the wound with wound closure strips or thin strips of tape (Figure 8).

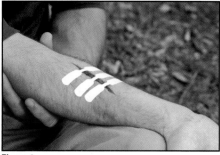

Figure 8

- If hair gets in the way of laceration closure, carefully clip it short. DO NOT shave.

- If using closure strips, apply one end of one strip to one side of the wound and another to the opposite side.

- Using the opposing strips as handles, you can pull the wound edges together, pulling the skin in as close as possible to where it should lie naturally.

■ Apply a thin layer of antibiotic ointment or a microthin (transparent) film dressing. DO NOT use an ointment with a microthin film dressing.

■ Cover the wound with a sterile dressing and bandage. If possible, the dressing should completely cover the wound and extend ½ inch beyond the wound's edge.

■ Remove rings or anything that could cut off circulation if swelling occurs.

■ Check bandages often.

■ If possible, change the dressing daily. Microthin film dressings may be left in place until healing is complete.

NOTE ■ Wounds gaping more than ½ inch should not be closed in the field but instead evacuated for closure by a health care provider.

■ Large dirty wounds; wounds that expose bones, tendons or ligaments; and wounds caused by animal bites should be left open. These are difficult to clean well enough to prevent infection.

■ Exceptionally dirty wounds should be packed open with sterile gauze and covered with dry gauze to allow them to drain until a health care provider can be consulted.

Abrasions

Abrasions are shallow and often dirty wounds that occur when some skin has been scraped away (Figure 9). They are often infected and can be painful.

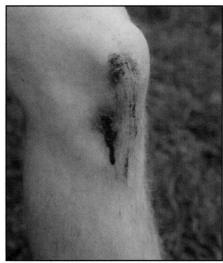

Figure 9

To give CARE:

- If cared for *within* 10 minutes, apply a thick layer of antibiotic ointment and cover with a sterile dressing, then bandage.
- If cared for *after* 10 minutes or there are items (e.g., sand, pebbles) in the wound:
  - Scrub the abrasion clean with a gauze pad or a clean, soft cloth and soap and water.
  - Follow scrubbing with irrigation or rinsing.
  - Apply a thin layer of antibiotic ointment and cover with a dressing and bandage.

Friction Blisters

To give CARE:

- Clean around the site thoroughly.
- Sterilize the point of a needle or knife to open the blister wide.
- If possible, leave the roof (separated skin layer) of the blister intact to ease discomfort and speed healing.
- Wash with soap and water.
- If the roof has been rubbed away, care for as an open wound.

- In all cases, apply a dressing that limits friction.
  - If available, use a commercial product or improvise with duct tape and gauze.
  - Building a "donut" by cutting a hole in the center of a rounded piece of moleskin (Figure 10) or improvising something similar separates irritated skin from friction.
  - Center the blister site in the hole and fill the hole with ointment, preferably antibiotic ointment.
  - Tape the moleskin or put another strip of moleskin on top of the donut to keep the ointment in place (Figure 11). This also prevents the blister from refilling with liquid.

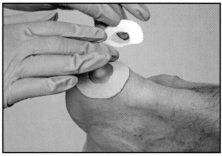

Figure 10

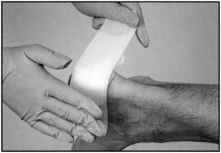

Figure 11

Chafing

Chafing occurs from excess friction, often in the groin area and between the thighs.

To give **CARE**:

- Apply a layer of lubricating oil or ointment (e.g., petroleum jelly or cooking oil) or fragrance-free baby powder or cornstarch.

Ear Problems

To give **CARE**:

For objects lodged in the ear:

- DO NOT use force to remove the object.
- If it is small, attempt to rinse it out with water by flooding and draining the ear canal.
  - For insects, use cooking oil instead of water.

For ear infections:

When **CHECK**ing the patient, look, listen and feel for:

- Pain when the ear is pulled on.
- Vertigo (dizziness).

To give **CARE**:

- Rinse the ear daily with a solution of 50 percent water and 50 percent alcohol or vinegar.
- Seek medical help if pain persists.

Nosebleeds

To give **CARE**:

- Have the patient sit down, lean forward and pinch the meaty part of the nose, just below the bridge, firmly shut (Figure 12). You may have to do this if the patient is unable.

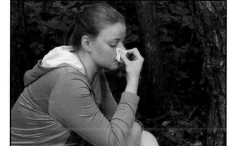

Figure 12

- Hold or have the patient hold the nose shut for 10 minutes.
- If bleeding persists, have the patient continue pinching the nose shut for another 10 minutes and repeat until bleeding stops.
- Care for continued bleeding by packing the nostrils gently with gauze soaked with antibiotic ointment or a decongestant nasal spray.
- If the patient suffered a blow to the nose that caused a deformity, care for the injury with cold packs.
- Ask the patient not to blow his or her nose for 10 days because this could restart bleeding.
- Have the patient seek professional help within 10 days if the nose was deformed by trauma.

> **NOTE** Blood running down the throat when leaning forward may indicate a serious nosebleed. The patient will need rapid evacuation and a health care provider's attention.

Teeth Problems

⊚ To give CARE:

For a cavity or missing filling:

- Rinse the area clean.
- Apply a drop of oil of cloves (eugenol) to ease the pain.
- Make a temporary filling by mixing zinc powder oxide and eugenol or use candle wax, ski wax or sugarless gum.
- To hold a dislodged crown back in place, use temporary filling material or a commercial dental adhesive product (e.g., Fixadent®).

For a knocked-out tooth:

- Bleeding can be controlled by biting down on a rolled gauze pad. Have the patient rinse his or her mouth out.
- Hold the tooth by the crown and avoid touching the root.
- Rinse the tooth with clean water. DO NOT scrub.
- Gently press the tooth back in the socket.
- If the tooth will not go back in, save it until the patient can get to a dentist.
- To store the loose tooth, have the patient hold it in his or her mouth, taking care not to swallow it.
- If the patient cannot hold the tooth in his or her mouth, ideally store the tooth in milk or a 0.9 percent saline solution.

For an infected tooth:

⊘ When CHECKing the patient, look, listen and feel for:

- Pain and swelling in the gum and cheek near the tooth.
- Possible discoloration of the gum.

⊚ To give CARE:

- Place cold packs on the cheek.
- If evacuation is delayed, have the patient rinse out his or her mouth several times a day with warm, salty water.
- Aspirin may help alleviate pain.

NOTE Evacuate the patient rapidly—GO FAST.

NOTE The patient should only take medication if he or she can swallow and has no known contraindications. Patients should read and follow all label or health care provider instructions. Check state and local regulations regarding use of prescription and over-the-counter medications.

Mosquito Bites

To give CARE:

- Care for with topical over-the-counter agents.
- To avoid creating open wounds that can become infected, DO NOT scratch.
- If flu-like symptoms develop within 2 weeks of a mosquito bite, see a health care provider for evaluation.

Tick Bites

To give CARE:

- Remove the tick immediately.
  - Grasp the tick as close to the skin as possible, perpendicular to its long axis and pull it out slowly using tweezers or gloved fingers.
- Wash the bite area and apply antibiotic ointment to prevent infection.
- Wash your hands.
- If flu-like symptoms develop within 2 weeks of a tick bite, see a health care provider for evaluation.
- If the tick was attached for longer than 48 to 72 hours, the patient should see a health care provider upon returning home.

Bee or Wasp Stings

To give CARE:

- Carefully remove the stinger with tweezers or scrape it away from the skin using your fingernail or a plastic card (e.g., a credit card). Wasps do not lose their stinger. If you use tweezers, grasp the stinger, not the venom sac.
- Wash the site and cover it to keep the site clean.
- Apply cold to the area.

Snakebites

⊘ When **CHECK**ing the patient, look, listen and feel for:

- One or more fang marks, with or without bleeding.
- Localized pain.
- Swelling, possibly of the entire limb.
- Nausea, vomiting and tingling (signs of moderate envenomation [poisoning]).
- Shock, coma and paralysis (signs of severe poisoning).
- Necrosis (tissue death) at site.

⊘ To give **CARE**:

- Keep the patient physically and emotionally calm.
- Gently wash the bite site.
- Splint bitten extremities, keeping the bite site at approximately the level of the patient's heart.
- DO NOT cut, suck, apply a constricting band or apply cold to a bite from a pit viper (e.g., rattlesnake, copperhead or cotton mouth). For a bite from an elapid snake (e.g., coral snake), apply an elastic roller bandage after washing the wound.
- Go for help.
- Unless it is unavoidable, DO NOT allow the patient to walk.
- Have the snakebite evaluated by a health care provider.

> **NOTE** Care for snakebites as puncture wounds that might cause infections, including tetanus.

Wound Infection

⊘ When **CHECK**ing the patient, look, listen and feel for:

In mild infections:

- Pain, redness and swelling.
- Small amount of light-colored pus.

In serious infections:

- Increasing pain, redness and swelling.
- Increasing heat at the site.
- Foul-smelling pus that increases and grows darker in color.
- Appearance of red streaks just under the skin near the wound.
- Systemic fever.

⊙ To give CARE:

For mild infections:

■ Re-clean with soap and water and re-dress the wound.

■ Apply antibiotic ointment.

■ Monitor for signs of serious infection. For any large bruised areas, bites or poisoning incidences, outline the affected area in pen and indicate the time that the wound occurred to help you determine if the area is growing over time. Act early if signs of infection are seen.

For serious infections:

■ Re-clean the wound with water and apply antibiotic ointment.

■ Allow the wound to re-open and let it drain. Soak the wound in water as hot as the patient can tolerate.

■ Pack the wound with moist, sterile gauze to keep it draining.

■ Dress the surface of the wound with dry, sterile gauze.

■ Re-clean and repack the wound twice a day during an extended evacuation.

■ Monitor the wound closely.

⊙ CALLing for Help: Guidelines for Evacuation

■ Evacuate slowly—**GO SLOW**—anyone with a wound that cannot be closed in the field.

■ Evacuate rapidly—**GO FAST**—anyone with a wound that:
  ● Is heavily contaminated.
  ● Opens a joint space or body cavity.
  ● Involves tendons or ligaments.
  ● Was caused by an animal bite.
  ● Is deep and on the face.
  ● Involves an impalement.
  ● Was caused by a crushing injury.

■ Evacuate rapidly—**GO FAST**—anyone with an infected wound or skin infection that does not improve within 12 hours of care or that spreads to other parts of the body.

■ Evacuate rapidly—**GO FAST**—anyone with signs and symptoms of a serious infection.

■ If more than one patient breaks out in skin boils or abscesses, evacuate all rapidly and immediately seek advanced medical care. This may be a sign of group contamination with methicillin-resistant *Staphylococcus aureus* (MRSA), a serious staphylococcal infection.

Special
Situations

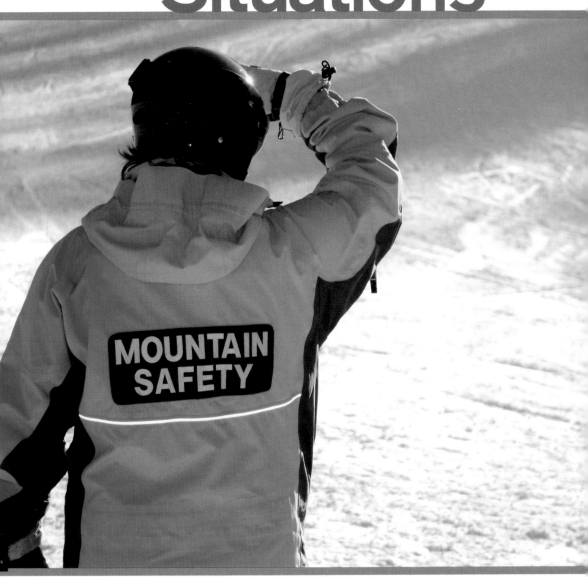

Abdominal Injuries and Illnesses

Giardia (Parasite)

⊘ When **CHECK**ing the patient, look, listen and feel for:

With acute infection:

- Diarrhea lasting 10 days or more.
- Foul-smelling stools and gas.
- Fatigue.
- Abdominal distention (swelling).

With chronic infection:

- Intermittent episodes of:
  - Mushy, foul-smelling stools.
  - Abdominal pain and distention.
  - Gas.
  - Loss of appetite.
  - Weight loss.
  - Fatigue.

♡ To give **CARE**:

- Care for persistent diarrhea. See Diarrhea.
- Have the patient examined by a health care provider as soon as possible.

Open Abdominal Injuries

⊘ When **CHECK**ing the patient, look, listen and feel for:

- Visible or protruding intestines.

To give CARE:

- DO NOT apply direct pressure.
- DO NOT attempt to push intestines back into the cavity.
- Remove clothing from around the wound.
- Apply moist, sterile dressings loosely over the wound (Figure 1).
- Cover dressings loosely with plastic wrap, if available. Foil or a plastic bag will also work.
- Give nothing by mouth.

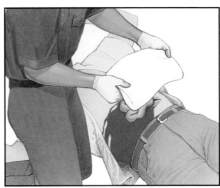

Figure 1

Closed Abdominal Injuries

When CHECKing the patient, look, listen and feel for:

- Mechanism of injury (e.g., blunt force) associated with closed abdominal injuries.
- Signs and symptoms of shock.
- Bruising.
- Abdominal rigidity or tenderness.
- Gradually increasing pulse.
- Pale skin.
- Nausea.

To give CARE:

- Closely observe the patient.
- Care for shock.
- Evacuate as soon as possible.
- Note quadrant of pain (Figure 2) and describe it on report form.

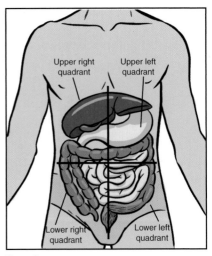

Upper right quadrant

Upper left quadrant

Lower right quadrant

Lower left quadrant

Figure 2

Asthma Attack

Asthma is a condition that narrows the air passages in the lungs and makes breathing difficult.

✅ When CHECKing the patient, look, listen and feel for:

- Coughing or wheezing.
- Trouble breathing.
- Shortness of breath.
- Rapid, shallow breathing.
- Inability to talk without stopping for a breath.
- Tightness in the chest.
- Feelings of fear or confusion.
- Sweating.

❤ To give CARE:

- Reassure the patient that you are going to help.
- Have the patient rest in a comfortable position.
- Administer oxygen, if trained.
- Assist the patient with or have the patient self-administer a prescribed inhaler (Figure 1).

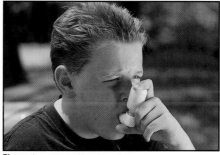

Figure 1

> **NOTE** The patient should only take medication if he or she has no known contraindications. Patients should read and follow all label or health care provider instructions. Check state and local regulations regarding use of prescription and over-the-counter medications.

- Help the patient sit up and rest in a position comfortable for breathing.
- Ensure that the prescription is in the patient's name and is prescribed for "quick relief" or "acute" attacks.

> **NOTE** Some inhalers contain long-acting, preventive medication that should not be used in an emergency.

- Ensure that the expiration date of the medication has not passed.
- Read and follow all instructions printed on the inhaler prior to administering the medication to the patient.
- Shake the inhaler.
- Remove the cover from the inhaler mouthpiece. Some inhalers have extension or spacer tubes that fit between the mouthpiece and the medication canister (Figure 2). If present, attach and use.

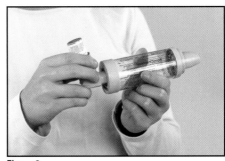

Figure 2

- Tell the patient to breathe out as much as possible.
- Have the patient place his or her lips tightly around the mouthpiece. The patient may use different techniques.
- As the patient breathes in slowly, administer the medication by quickly pressing down on the inhaler canister, or the patient may self-administer the medication.
    - The patient should continue a full, deep breath.
    - Tell the patient to try to hold his or her breath for a count of 10. When using an extension tube, have the patient take 5 to 6 deep breaths through the tube without holding his or her breath.
- Note the time of administration and any change in the patient's condition.
    - The medication may be repeated once after 1 to 2 minutes.

NOTE The medication may be repeated every 5 to 10 minutes thereafter as needed. These medications might take 5 to 15 minutes to reach full effectiveness.

- Stay with the patient and monitor his or her condition and give care for any other injuries. Have the patient rinse his or her mouth out with water.
- Care for shock. Keep the patient from getting chilled or overheated.

NOTE If a patient has an inhaler, you may assist with administration if you are trained to do so and local and state protocols allow.

CALLing for Help: Guidelines for Evacuation

- Evacuate rapidly—**GO FAST**—if breathing does not improve within 15 minutes.

Cold-Related Emergencies

Frostbite

Frostbite is the freezing of body parts exposed to the cold. Severity depends on the air temperature, length of exposure and the wind. Frostbite can cause the loss of fingers, hands, arms, toes, feet and legs.

⊘ When CHECKing the patient, look, listen and feel for:

- Numbness or lack of feeling in the affected area.
- Skin that appears waxy, is cold to the touch or is discolored (i.e., flushed, white, yellow or blue).
- Late stages which may include gangrene and black and leathery skin (Figure 1).

♥ To give CARE:

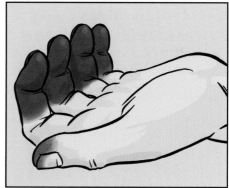

Figure 1

- Handle the area gently.
- Never rub an affected area. Rubbing causes further damage to soft tissues.
- Protect the patient from further exposure and give care for hypothermia. If hands are frostbitten, place them in armpit area or between thighs. If nose is frostbitten, cover with a hand.
- DO NOT attempt re-warming if there is a chance of re-freezing or help is more than 2 hours away.
- If you are in a remote area and close to a medical facility, slowly re-warm the frostbitten part by soaking it in water not warmer than 105°F (Figure 2). Keep the frostbitten part in the water until normal color returns and it feels warm.
- Loosely bandage the area with a dry, sterile dressing.

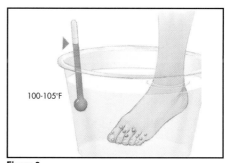

100-105°F

Figure 2

- If fingers or toes are frostbitten, place cotton or gauze between them (Figure 3).
- Do not break any blisters.

Immersion Foot

Immersion foot occurs when feet have been exposed to more than 12 hours of cold, wet conditions. If the person has experienced immersion foot before or does not have healthy feet, it can occur in as little as 3 hours. Tissues do not freeze, but there is nerve and circulatory damage.

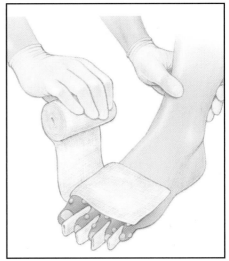

Figure 3

✓ When CHECKing the patient, look, listen and feel for:

- *Initial signs and symptoms:*
  - Swollen, cold, waxy feet
  - Peeling skin (Figure 4)
  - Reduced sensitivity to touch
  - Wooden feeling in feet
  - Delayed capillary refill time (nail beds stay white after you squeeze them)
- *After the foot warms up:*
  - Warm, dry, red skin
  - Pain
  - Increased sensitivity to cold
  - Blisters
  - Tingling or itching

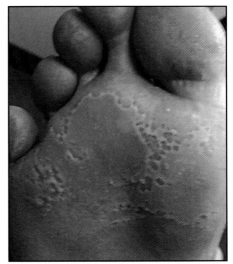

Figure 4

♡ To give CARE:

- Care for the affected part by applying warm packs or soaking in warm water (102° to 105° F) for approximately 5 minutes.
- Elevate the affected area.
- Clean and dry feet.
- Give plenty of fluids to drink.
- DO NOT allow the person to wear wet socks or shoes.
- Obtain medical assistance as soon as possible.

Confined Spaces

If a person becomes injured or ill in a confined space, you will need to take specific precautions before attempting to respond to the emergency. A *confined space* is any space that has limited access and is not intended for continuous human occupancy. At a worksite, a confined space would be large enough that an employee could enter and perform assigned work.

Examples of confined spaces include:

- Tunnels.
- Agricultural silos, grain bins and grain elevators.
- Underground vaults.
- Utility vaults for water, sewers or electrical power.
- Spaces that result from cave-ins.

In the wilderness or remote areas, examples of confined spaces include:

- Crevasses.
- Caves.
- Abandoned mines.
- Wells, culverts and cisterns that could contain water.

Rescues in confined spaces are usually for falls, explosions, asphyxia, medical problems or machinery entrapment.

⊘ CHECKing the Scene and the Resources and ⊙ CALLing for Help

When checking a confined space scene, determine if the situation is too dangerous for you to reach the injured or ill person safely. Examples of unsafe conditions include the presence of:

- Fire.
- Smoked-filled spaces.
- Poison gas or hazardous material (HAZMAT) markings.
- Possible natural or propane gas explosions.
- Collapsed or partially collapsed structures.
- Confined areas with no ventilation or fresh air.

Avoid entering areas that require special training and equipment (e.g., respirators, self-contained breathing apparatus [SCBA]).

Without entering the confined space, try to determine how many people are involved and whether there are any hazards present. Next, call for help and be as specific as possible about the situation, so the appropriate personnel can be dispatched. Establish a safe perimeter around the area, preventing anyone from entering. Do not enter the scene unless you are sure it is safe. When able, assist in the rescue and offer medical assistance if appropriate.

> **NOTE** Avoid the use of oxygen combined with the use of an automated external defibrillator (AED) in a confined space.

Diabetic Emergency

People with diabetes sometimes become ill because there is too much or too little sugar in their blood.

⊘ When **CHECK**ing the patient, look, listen and feel for:
- A medical identification (ID) tag, bracelet or necklace.
- Light-headedness, dizziness, confusion or weakness.
- Irregular breathing.
- Irregular pulse (rapid or weak).
- Feeling or looking ill.
- Changes in levels of responsiveness (LOR).
- Gradual or rapid onset of confusion or disorientation.
- Dry, red skin.
- Pale, moist skin.

⊚ To give **CARE:**
- Reassure the patient that you are going to help.
- If the patient is alert and can safely swallow food or fluids and is known to have diabetes, give sugar (e.g., fruit juices, non-diet soft drinks, sugar packets, cake decorating gel, candy, oral glucose).
- Monitor the patient for changes in consciousness.
- Have the patient check his or her own sugar level, if he or she knows how.

- If the patient has insulin, you can get it for the patient. The patient must self-administer the insulin.
- If the patient is unconscious:
  - DO NOT give anything to eat or drink.
  - Care for the conditions you find.

⊙ CALLing for Help: Guidelines for Evacuation

- Evacuate rapidly–**GO FAST**–anyone who does not feel better in about 5 minutes.
- Evacuate rapidly–**GO FAST**–anyone who is unconscious.

Emergency and Non-Emergency Moves

One of the most dangerous threats to a seriously injured person is unnecessary movement. Moving a seriously injured person can cause additional injury and pain and make the recovery more difficult. You should move a person only in the following three situations:

- When you are faced with immediate danger (e.g., fire).
- When you must get to another person who may have a more serious injury or illness.
- When you must move the person to give proper care.

If you must move the person for one of these reasons, you must quickly decide how to do so. Carefully consider your safety and the safety of the injured person.

To avoid hurting yourself or the injured person, use your legs, not your back, when you bend. Bend at the knees and hips and avoid twisting your body. Walk forward when possible, taking small steps and looking where you are going. Avoid twisting or bending anyone who you think has a possible head, neck or back injury. If you cannot move a person safely, do not move the person.

Walking Assist

To help a patient who needs help walking to safety:

1. Place the patient's arm around your shoulders or waist, depending on his or her size, and hold it in place with one hand.
2. Support the patient with your other hand around the patient's waist (Figure 1).
3. Move the patient to safety.

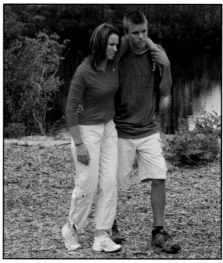

Figure 1

Another person, if present, can support the patient in the same way on the other side.

Pack-Strap Carry

To move either a conscious or an unconscious patient when you do not suspect a head, neck or back injury:

1. Position yourself in front of the patient with your back to the patient's front.
2. Place the patient's arms over your shoulders and cross them in front of your neck, then grasp the patient's wrists.
3. Lean forward slightly and pull the patient onto your back (Figure 2). To do this, you may have to kneel close to the ground. Then, when you lift, use the power in your legs to get up and move.
4. Move the patient to safety.

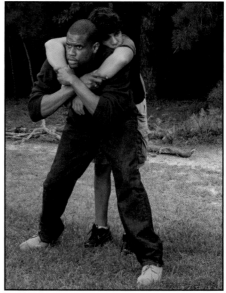

Figure 2

Two-Person Seat Carry

To carry a patient who cannot walk and
who you do not think has a head, neck
or back injury:

1. Put one arm under the patient's
   thighs and the other across the
   patient's back, under his or her arms.
2. Interlock your arms with another
   person's arms under the patient's
   legs and across the patient's back.
3. Lift the patient in the "seat" formed
   by your interlocked arms (Figure 3).
4. Move the patient to safety.

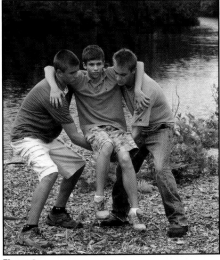

Figure 3

Clothes Drag

To move a patient who may have a
head, neck or back injury:

1. Gather the patient's clothing behind
   his or her neck. While moving the
   patient, cradle the head with his or
   her clothes and your hands.
2. Pull the patient to safety (Figure 4).

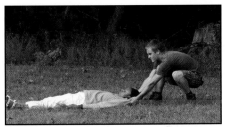

Figure 4

Blanket Drag

To move a patient in an emergency
situation when equipment is limited:

1. Keep the patient between you and
   the blanket.
2. Gather half the blanket and place it
   against the patient's side.
3. Roll the patient toward you as a unit.
4. Reach over the patient and place the
   blanket under the patient.
5. Roll the patient onto the blanket.
6. Gather the blanket at the head and move the patient to safety (Figure 5).

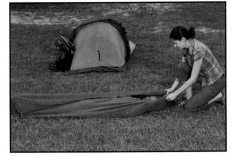

Figure 5

Foot Drag

To move a patient who is too large to
carry or otherwise move:

1. Firmly grasp the patient's ankles and
   move backward (Figure 6).
2. Pull the patient in a straight line and
   be careful not to bump his or her
   head.

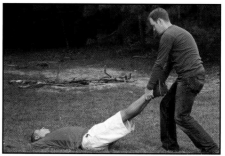

Figure 6

Stretchers

A stretcher (litter) can be used to move a patient a short distance to a better site
for giving care. A stretcher can also be used to transport an injured or ill patient
a longer distance. Choose one of the following methods based on the patient's
injuries:

- Blanket stretcher
- Rope stretcher
- Coat stretcher
- Improvised sled
- Pack frame stretcher

Assess what equipment you have to improvise a stretcher.

- Rope
- Backpack
- Pack frame and pole
- Tent fly
- Webbing band
- Tent poles or wooden poles
- Toboggan or ski sled
- Plastic tarp

A good stretcher:

- Is stable.
- Can be tipped over without the patient falling out.
- Keeps the patient safe and does not make the patient's injuries worse.
- Will not injure the person carrying it.
- Is strong enough to deal with the terrain.

- Is strong enough to deal with the movement it will be subjected to.
- Makes the person feel safe and comfortable (within reason).
- Can be controlled from both ends at the same time.

When carrying a stretcher, make sure:
- The patient in the stretcher is wearing eye protection so debris does not get into his or her eyes.
- The patient's head is pointing uphill.
- There are three people on each side to carry the stretcher over rough or steep terrain, plus one leader and two people with ropes to control the rate of descent or uphill movement.

Emergency Childbirth

To give CARE:

If a woman is giving birth:
- Talk with the woman to help her stay calm.
- Place layers of newspaper covered with layers of linens, towels or blankets under the woman.
- Control the scene so that the woman will have privacy.
- Position her on her back with knees bent, feet flat and legs spread wide apart.
- Remember, the woman delivers the baby, so be patient and let it happen naturally.
- Keep the baby warm.

Caution:
- Do not let the woman get up or leave to find a bathroom. (Most women have a desire to use the restroom.)
- Do not hold her knees together; this will not slow the birth process and may complicate the birth or harm the baby.
- Do not place your fingers in the vagina for any reason.
- Do not pull on the baby.

CALLing for Help: Guidelines for Evacuation
- Evacuate slowly—**GO SLOW**—if possible. Give advanced medical personnel the woman's name, age, expected due date, how long she has been having labor pains and if this is her first child.

Eye, Mouth and Lip Injuries

Eye Injuries

⊚ To give CARE:

- If an eye is burned by a chemical, flush the affected eye with large amounts of water for at least 20 minutes.
- Care for open and closed wounds around the eye as you would for any other soft tissue injury.
- DO NOT put direct pressure on the eyeball.
- Remember that *all* eye injuries should be examined by a health care provider.
- If foreign bodies get in the eye (e.g., dust), tell the patient *not* to rub the eyes. DO NOT touch the eye.
  - Have the patient blink several times.
  - If the object is visible on the lower eyelid, pull the eyelid down and try to remove the object with the corner of a sterile gauze pad. Be careful *not* to touch the eyeball.
  - Gently flush the eye with irrigation, saline solution or water.
  - After irrigating, if the object is visible on the upper eyelid, gently roll the upper eyelid back over a cotton swab and attempt to remove the object with the corner of a sterile gauze pad, being careful *not* to touch the eyeball.
  - If the object remains, the patient should receive advanced medical care.
  - Cover the injured eye with an eye pad/shield.
- If an object is impaled in the eye, DO NOT attempt to remove it.
  - Keep the patient on his or her back and have someone perform manual stabilization.
  - Stabilize the object by encircling the eye with a gauze dressing or soft sterile cloth, being careful not to apply any pressure to the area.
  - Position bulky dressings around the impaled object (e.g., roller gauze) and then cover it with a shield (e.g., a paper cup). DO NOT use Styrofoam®-type materials, as small particles can break off and get into the eye. The shield should not touch the object.

- Bandage the shield and dressing in place with a self-adhering bandage and roller bandage covering the patient's injured eye to keep the object stable and minimize movement.
- Comfort and reassure the patient.
- Do not leave the patient unattended.

Mouth Injuries

⊙ To give CARE:

- Make sure the person is able to breathe as injuries to the mouth may cause breathing problems if blood or loose teeth obstruct the airway.
- If the patient is bleeding from the mouth and you do not suspect a serious head, neck or spinal injury, place the patient in a seated position with the head tilted slightly forward.
- If this position is not possible, place the patient on his or her side in the recovery position to allow blood to drain from the mouth.

Lip Injuries

⊙ To give CARE:

- Place a rolled dressing between the lip and the gum.
- Place another dressing on the outer surface of the lip.
- If the tongue is bleeding, apply a dressing and direct pressure.
- Apply cold to the lips or tongue to reduce swelling and ease pain.

Poisoning

A poison is any substance that causes injury, illness or death if it enters the body. A person can be poisoned by swallowing poison, breathing it, absorbing it through the skin and having it injected into the body.

⊘ When CHECKing the patient, look, listen and feel for:

- Trouble breathing.
- Nausea, vomiting and/or diarrhea.
- Chest or stomach pain.
- Sweating.
- Changes in alertness.
- Seizures.
- Burns around the lips or tongue or on the skin.
- Open or spilled containers.
- Overturned or damaged plants.
- Unusual odors, flames and/or smoke.
- Headache.
- Dizziness.
- Exposure to plants, such as poison ivy (Figure 1, A), poison sumac (Figure 1, B) or poison oak (Figure 1, C).

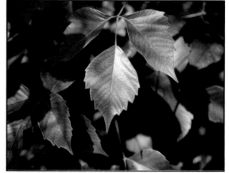

Figure 1A

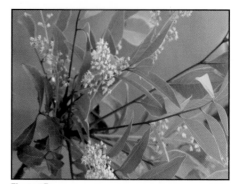

Figure 1B

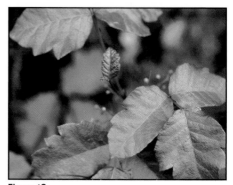

Figure 1C

To give **CARE**:

- Look for any containers that may contain a harmful or poisonous substance.
- If necessary, move the patient to safety, away from the source of the poison.
- Check the patient's level of responsiveness (LOR), movement and breathing.
- Reassure the patient that you are going to help.
- If you suspect a conscious patient has been poisoned and no immediate life-threatening condition is found and you have access to a phone, call the National Poison Control Center (PCC) hotline at 800-222-1222.
- DO NOT give the patient anything to eat or drink unless directed to do so by PCC or emergency medical services (EMS) personnel.
- If you suspect a patient has swallowed a poison, try to find out the type of poison, how much was taken and when it was taken.
- If the patient vomits, position him or her in a recovery position.

Poisonous Plants

To give **CARE**:

- Reassure the patient that you are going to help.
- If skin is exposed, immediately wash the affected area thoroughly with soap and water (wear disposable gloves).
- If a rash or open sores develop, apply a paste of baking soda and water several times a day to reduce discomfort.
- Apply lotions (e.g., Caladryl™) which may help soothe the area, if the patient has no known contraindications.
- Wash clothing exposed to plant oils with soap. Wash your hands thoroughly after handling exposed clothing.

Scorpion Stings and Spider Bites

To give **CARE**:

If someone has been stung by a scorpion or bitten by a black widow spider or brown recluse spider:

- Wash the wound.
- Apply a cold pack to the site.

- If it is available, give the person antivenin (a medication that blocks the effects of poisonous venom).
- If signs of allergic reaction or anaphylaxis develop, treat with antihistamines or epinephrine, if the patient has an auto-injector. Life-threatening signs and symptoms require evacuation to advanced medical care. See Allergies and Anaphylaxis.

Animal Bites

⊙ To give CARE:
- Control bleeding first if the wound is bleeding seriously.
- Do not clean serious wounds; the wound will be cleaned at a medical facility.
- Wash minor wounds with soap and water.
- Control any bleeding.
- Apply an antibiotic ointment and a dressing.
- Watch for signs of infection.

Marine Life Stings

⊙ To give CARE:
- If signs of allergic reaction or anaphylaxis develop, treat with antihistamines, or if the patient has an auto-injector, treat with epinephrine. Life-threatening signs and symptoms require evacuation to advanced medical care. See Allergies and Anaphylaxis.

For a jellyfish sting:
- Remove stingers.
- Soak the area in vinegar.

For a stingray sting:
- Immobilize the area.
- Soak the area in non-scalding hot water until pain goes away.
- Clean and bandage the wound.
- Watch for signs of infection.

⊚ CALLing for Help: Guidelines for Evacuation

- Evacuate slowly–**GO SLOW**–anyone with conditions that are worsening or affect large areas of the body or face.
- Evacuate rapidly–**GO FAST**–anyone who is unconscious, or if there is a change in the level of responsiveness (LOR) or another life-threatening condition is present. Care for any life-threatening conditions, if found.
- Evacuate rapidly–**GO FAST**–anyone who exhibits a severe reaction to a sting or bite by bugs or marine life.
- Evacuate rapidly–**GO FAST**–anyone with a wound that is bleeding seriously from an animal bite or if you suspect the animal might have rabies.

Seizures

When the normal functions of the brain are disrupted by injury, disease, fever, poisoning or infection, the electrical activity of the brain becomes irregular. The irregularity can cause a loss of body control, known as *seizure*.

Seizures may be caused by a condition called *epilepsy*, which is usually controllable with medication. Some children and infants have seizures that are caused by a sudden high fever.

⊘ When **CHECK**ing the patient, look, listen and feel for:

- Unusual sensation or feeling such as a visual hallucination (patient is experiencing an aura).
- Irregular or no breathing.
- Drooling.
- Upward rolling of the eyes.
- Rigid body.
- Sudden, uncontrollable, rhythmic muscle contractions (convulsions) (Figure 1).
- Decreased level of responsiveness (LOR).
- Loss of bladder or bowel control.

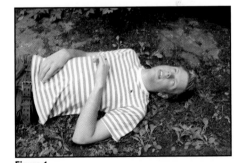

Figure 1

⦿ To give CARE:

- Reassure the patient that you are going to help.
- Remove nearby objects that might cause injury.
- Protect the patient's head by placing a thinly folded towel or clothing beneath it (Figure 2). DO NOT restrict the airway doing so.

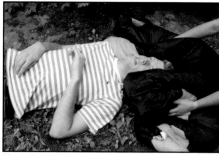

Figure 2

- DO NOT hold or restrain the patient.
- DO NOT place anything between the patient's teeth.
- Place the patient on his or her side to drain fluids from the mouth.
- If the seizure was caused by a sudden rise in body temperature, loosen clothing and fan the patient. DO NOT immerse in cold water or use rubbing alcohol to cool.
- When the seizure is over, be sure that the patient's airway is open and check for breathing and injuries.
- Comfort and stay with the patient until he or she is fully conscious.

⦿ CALLing for Help: Guidelines for Evacuation

- Evacuate rapidly—**GO FAST**—anyone who has a seizure that lasts more than a few minutes or has repeated seizures.
- Evacuate rapidly—**GO FAST**—anyone who is pregnant or has diabetes and has a seizure.
- Evacuate rapidly—**GO FAST**—anyone who has a seizure in the water or who does not regain responsiveness following a seizure.

Snow Blindness

Snow blindness is a radiation burn (sunburn) of the eye. It is named for the reflection off snow, but can also happen due to bright sunlight. After giving care, the patient may be able to self-evacuate with help. Improvised sunglasses (e.g., cardboard with narrow slit) may aid the patient.

♥ To give CARE:

- Stop the burning by wearing sunglasses or covering eyes.
- Have the patient remove contact lenses and rest.
- If the patient can swallow and has no known contraindications, the patient can self-administer aspirin.

> **NOTE** The patient should only take medication if he or she can swallow and has no known contraindications. Patients should read and follow all label or health care provider instructions. Check state and local regulations regarding use of prescription and over-the-counter medications.

Stroke

Internal injury to the brain can be a stroke—with catastrophic results. A stroke is caused when blood flow to a part of the brain is cut off or when there is bleeding into the brain.

◎ When **CHECK**ing the patient:

- Use **FAST** to determine if the person has had a stroke:
  - **FACE**—Weakness on one side of the face
    - Ask the person to smile (Figure 1).
  - **ARM**—Weakness or numbness of one arm
    - Ask the person to raise both arms (Figure 2).
  - **SPEECH**—Slurred speech or trouble getting words out
    - Ask the person to speak a simple sentence.
  - **TIME**—Note the time that the signs and symptoms were first observed.

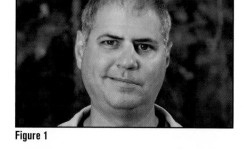

Figure 1

♥ To give **CARE**:

- Note the time that that signs and symptoms began.
- Monitor and care for the ABCDEs.
  - If the patient is unconscious, make sure he or she has an open airway and care for life-threatening conditions.
  - If fluid or vomit is in the patient's mouth, turn him or her on one side to allow fluids to drain.

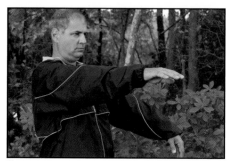

Figure 2

NOTE   Evacuate the patient rapidly—**GO FAST**—as this is a life-threatening condition.

Wound Care

Avulsion

Avulsion is an injury in which a portion of the skin, and sometimes other soft tissue, is partially or completely torn away.

To give **CARE**:

- Control external bleeding.
- Never remove the portion of the skin or soft tissue.
- Care for it as you would an open wound, stabilizing the part.

Amputation

Amputation is the complete removal or severing of an external body part.

To give **CARE**:

- Control external bleeding.
- If the amputation is incomplete, never remove the portion of the skin or soft tissue.
- If the body part is completely severed, once it has been found, wrap it in sterile gauze, moistened in sterile saline if available.
- Place it in a plastic bag and label it with the patient's name and the time and date it was placed in the bag.
- Keep the bag cool by placing it in a larger bag or container of an ice and water slurry, *not* on ice alone and *not* on dry ice.
- Transfer the bag to the advanced medical care transporting the patient to the hospital.

CALLing for Help: Guidelines for Evacuation

- Evacuate slowly–**GO SLOW**–anyone with an avulsion.
- Evacuate rapidly–**GO FAST**–anyone with an amputation.

Index